EASY
SLEEP

EASY SLEEP

JOHN J. GNAP, M.D.

with
Nancy Flaster

STEIN AND DAY/*Publishers*/New York

First Published in 1978
Copyright © 1978 by John J. Gnap, M.D. and Nancy Flaster
All rights reserved
Designed by Jared Pratt
Printed in the United States of America
Stein and Day/*Publishers*/Scarborough House,
Briarcliff Manor, N.Y. 10510

Library of Congress Cataloging in Publication Data

Gnap, John.
    Easy Sleep.

    Includes index.
       1.   Insomnia.   2.   Behavior modification.
    3.   Hypnotism—Therapeutic use.   I.   Flaster, Nancy,
    joint author.   II.   Title.
    RC548.G57   616.8'49   77-20879
    ISBN 0-8128-2435-0

To Jean Gnap
and
Samuel L. Flaster, M.D.

Acknowledgements

It is with respect and gratitude that I acknowledge the many patients who have taught me so much. Although their names do not appear in this book, none are anonymous to me.

I am also grateful to Marie Novak, Dr. John Gersack, Dr. Peter Lofendo, Edward Massura, and Richard Fisk for their advice and encouragement; to Jackie Calamos for typing the manuscript; to Marlene Chocola for secretarial assistance; and to Hubert Persoon for his electronics expertise and friendship. Special thanks also to Julietta S. Garcenila for her patience and support; to Rose Yeager and Lillian Flaster for reading the manuscript and offering valuable suggestions; to Sadie Markheim for her ongoing confidence; and to the Northbrook Public Library for its immeasurable aid.

Finally, my most profound gratitude goes to Jean Hazlehurst for her contributions to program administration and development; for her immeasurable assistance in preparing this book; and for her 10 years of unceasing dedication and understanding.

CONTENTS

CONTENTS

INTRODUCTION

The audience of physicians, nurses, and other health professionals gathered in the medical conference room to hear about the latest advances in sleep therapy. The speaker was a psychiatrist who specialized in the treatment of sleep disorders.

After a lengthy discussion on brain waves, biochemistry, rare pathological sleep disturbances, and the pros and cons of various drugs, the psychiatrist addressed himself to the most common sleep problem of them all—insomnia.

"The insomniac," he advised, "should be treated with reassurance since his problem is usually a symptom of psychological distress. To enhance sleep, I recommend walking a mile, eating a protein meal, taking a warm bath, reading a dull book, or having sex ... which is better than sleeping anyway."

The laughter that ensued showed that most of those present did not consider insomnia to be all that serious.

And relatively speaking, they're correct—insomnia poses no direct threat to your life. The effects of insomnia, like the effects of headaches, tend to make their mark on the quality more than the quantity of life.

Thus, while insomnia may not be statistically significant on the morbidity and mortality charts, it can definitely be personally significant to you. Frequent sleep problems can affect your productivity, your emotional well-being, your interpersonal relationships, your work, your play, and your zest for living. Even an occasional sleep problem can at times be devastating, particularly if it happens to occur the night before an exam, a job interview, or an important tennis match.

Unfortunately, the "cures" offered to insomniacs—the warm baths, mile-walks, medications, and the hundreds of other soporific formulas—seldom provide more than transient relief at best. Even well-intentioned admonitions such as, "Stop worrying so much" or "Don't think so much," are largely irrelevant. We all know that such advice is a lot easier said than done. And as for "reassurance" as a method of treatment, it may be comforting to know that your sleep problem isn't life-threatening; but reassurance in no way teaches you how to solve your sleep dilemma.

What about substituting sex for sleep? Anyone who hasn't had a good night's sleep for a while might feel just a bit too fatigued to take on sex as a permanent sleep substitute. When insomniacs utter the classic line, "Gee, I'm sorry, but I'm just too tired," they're probably speaking the truth. But who would believe them? Their excuse sounds about as credible as that other classic line: "Sorry, I have a headache." (By the way, those who advocate sexual activity *as a cure* for insomnia don't know much about insomnia. What they *do* know is that *they* fall asleep after *they* engage in sexual activity. But not everyone reacts that way. Furthermore, for most people, the idea of engaging in love-making for the therapeutic purpose of getting to sleep is somehow inapt.) In any case, sex is sex, and sleep is sleep.

Sleep . . . Easy Sleep . . . efficient sleep. The way to get it and keep it is through self-direction. Self-directed sleep does not rely on sex or food or pills or exercise or any other external devices to put you to sleep. Self-directed sleep relies only on you—you will be the one putting yourself to efficient and rejuvenating sleep. You will be the one turning sleep on and off at your own direction. That's Easy Sleep.

To actually gain control of your sleeping/waking processes may sound like a feat requiring the discipline of a guru. However, it actually requires less discipline than walking a mile every day or drinking a glass of warm milk every night. As a matter of fact, if you can *read* this book— if you can *understand* the printed word, you have all the necessary prerequisites for becoming an Easy Sleeper.

What does the Easy Sleep method entail?

First, that you gain a new understanding of sleep and your own sleeping problem.

Second, that you do a little planning so you'll feel more energetic during the day.

Third, that you practice a simple concentration technique in bed before you go to sleep.

I realize that when you pick up a "how-to" book, your natural inclination is to skip over explanatory chapters and turn straight to the "what-to-do" chapters. Thus, it would come as no surprise to me if you were now thinking: "Don't bother me with the 'whys' and 'wherefores' and 'new understanding.' Just give me the answers."

It has been my experience in more than 10 years of medical practice that telling a patient *what to do* is simply not enough. During my early years as a family practitioner, I told numerous patients *what to do:* "Follow this diet"; "Don't smoke so much"; "Don't drink so much"; "Don't work so hard"; "Relax more—you're too tense"; "Don't be so hard on yourself." However, when I saw that most patients apparently could not follow such advice, I came to realize how redundant my advice really was. *The patients already knew* what they *ought* to do.

What they did not know was *how* to do what *they needed to do.* I then began to teach patients how to use relaxation and concentration techniques in conjunction with their regular medical treatment. Results improved, but not with any consistency. Something was missing.

The missing element turned out to be *understanding.* Patients needed to understand how the relaxation and concentration techniques worked. They wanted to know how their use of the techniques would help them to make a change. As I started offering them a simplified educational component, their results improved dramatically. Not only did they understand why and how the techniques worked, but they also developed a *sense of self-direction* regarding their use of the techniques. *They were the ones* effecting changes in their systems. They no longer had the sense that something was being done *to them.*

In treating a variety of behavioral, emotional, and organic problems, I soon noticed that one of the earliest signs of a patient's progress was his improved ability to sleep. Although insomnia was not necessarily the patient's primary complaint, even as a secondary complaint, it was quickly and easily remedied. As I began to see more and more patients with primary complaints of insomnia, I found that the results of using a concentration technique in conjunction with an educational component were continuously positive and gratifying, for the patients as well as for me.

Based on my experience, I have concluded that if a patient is instructed to use a concentration technique to solve his sleep problem, he must also understand how and why the technique works. He must begin to expect the technique to work. The way to develop that kind of expectation is through understanding, education, and rational consideration. It's all got to make sense if it's going to work.

The first portion of this book, therefore, offers you some new insights and practical information so you can begin to expect the Easy Sleep technique to work for you. Even if all your previous attempts at solving your insomnia problems have failed, you will soon learn how it is possible and feasible to direct a desirable change in your sleep pattern. But, *you must first understand* what it is you're directing and changing. Then, you can easily implement the practice and maintenance techniques delineated in the latter portions of the book.

Once you have become adept at using the tools of self-directed sleep, you'll be able to apply your skills to a variety of potentially disruptive sleeping situations (such as the problems posed by jet travel across time zones, noisy neighbors, transient discomfort, anticipation when the "big day" is tomorrow). Toward the end of this book, you will find hints and suggestions for handling these common "sleep spoilers."

As you learn about Easy Sleep, you may notice that I have not devoted a great deal of space to the work being done by sleep researchers in laboratories across the country. Although I have a great deal of respect for the extraordinary work being conducted by these scientists, I do not believe these studies have an immediate practical application for the troubled sleeper. Printouts from EEGs (electroencephalographs), monitoring devices for rapid eye movements (REM), equipment for measuring muscular activity (EMG)—these may be significant from a scientific point of view. But for the insomniac, all the research data in the world in no way teaches you *how* to get a good night's sleep.

The purpose of this book is not to awe you with the physiologic mysteries of sleep. The purpose is to offer you what you'll need to know to get the kind of sleep you want.

In this book, I make one other noticeable departure from what is commonly written about sleep. Among the majority of health professionals, the consensus of opinion seems to be that most of our common sleep problems (and that means insomnia!) are more "mental" than "physical"— more "all in our minds" than "real." Or as the distinguished psychiatrist said to his audience: "Insomnia . . . is usually a symptom of psychological distress." (. . . And we know what that means!)

While it's undoubtedly true that emotional distress, anxiety, depression, tension, and other feelings are often the partners of insomnia, it is this book's contention that your feelings are *as physical* as your heartbeats—that what's in your head is real—that mind *is* matter.

In this book you'll learn that mental activities are *brain activities*. And your brain, through its *real*, electrochemical energy, integrates and facilitates all of your life's functions.

This book will show you how to go right to the core of your sleep problem—to actually *solve* the problem. Since the problem is in your brain, the solution is there also. Through the Easy Sleep method, you will discover how you can change a "can't sleep" habit recording on your brain, and how you can replace that old, undesirable recording with a new "can sleep" habit recording.

The basic tool for making that change is the Easy Sleep concentration technique—a simple procedure involving relaxation, concentration, and imagination. These three activities will come to mean something new to you as you gain an understanding of their tangible roles in harnessing your brain's energy and directing it to where you want it to go.

Through your new understanding, your practice, and some complementary daytime planning, your ability to sleep efficiently and awaken feeling refreshed will move into the realm of your own control. And once you've got it there—it's even easier to keep it.

EASY
SLEEP

The approach used in this book has been designed primarily for those who are troubled by common, uncomplicated insomnia. However, those whose sleep problems are complicated by other medical conditions can also derive significant benefits from using this book in conjunction with adequate medical care.

J.J.G.

1.

INSOMNIA: WHAT IT IS ... AND WHAT IT ISN'T

You toss ... you turn ... you get up and walk around the house ... you get back in bed ... you turn off the lights ... you turn on the lights ... you try reading a book ... you head for the refrigerator or medicine chest ... you pop something into your mouth (a pill, sandwich, bowl of ice cream, glass of milk, anything!) ... you get back in bed ... you toss ... you turn ... on go the lights ... and there goes the night. A night lost to insomnia.

No matter how many nights you've lost to insomnia or how many days you've dragged yourself around due to poor sleep, there is a way you can get the kind of sleep you want and need. The purpose of this book is to show you the way. In these pages, what you'll learn is something most people have never considered possible; that is, *you will learn how to produce sleep willfully and consciously at your own direction.*

This book's self-directed approach to sleep is distinctly different from other insomnia remedies. For all other remedies operate on the assumption that the sleeping/waking process is beyond your direct, voluntary control. "Take this!" "Try this!" "Do this!" they proclaim, and *hopefully* sleep will *overtake you.* But if sleep doesn't overtake you after you've taken the pills or walked around the block or had your warm baths or whatever, you're pretty much helpless to do anything about your predicament.

Through the Easy Sleep approach, you will never have to be in that helpless position again. YOU will be the one making sleep happen at your own direction. You will learn quickly how to sleep *when, where,* and *how much* YOU CHOOSE TO. You will also learn how to get the kind of sleep that refreshes and energizes you for the next day.

All you'll need to become an Easy Sleeper is to understand the concepts described in this book, to practice a simple, three-step concentration technique a few minutes each night before you want to go to sleep, and to do a little daytime planning. *Understanding, Practice;* and *Planning* —that's all it takes. And what you'll get is a reasonable, pleasant, and effective cure for one of the most frustrating ailments known to man and woman: insomnia.

Multitudes of "Sole Survivors"

There's something horrible about being awake when it seems like everyone else in the world is sleeping. Sometimes I look out my window to see if anyone else's lights are on. But even if I spot a few lights here and there, I always assume *they* are either having a wild party or are studying for an exam. *They* want to be up. I'm the only one who doesn't want to be up. After a while, I feel like a nervous wreck . . . it's like the world has come to an end and I'm the sole survivor.

Elaine, 28, a former insomniac

Anyone who has ever spent a night like Elaine's in frustrating wakefulness can tell you that insomnia is a lonely feeling. You can indeed feel like the "sole survivor" on the planet—unless, of course, you happen to run into another "sole survivor." Witness this exchange between two friends:

"I'm really wiped out today. I just couldn't sleep last night." "I wish I'd known . . . I would have called you. I was up tossing and turning 'til the crack of dawn."

If all of insomnia's "survivors" ever formed a fellowship to give each other emotional support, the comforting calls between members of the club would tie up telephone circuits permanently.

According to surveys, an estimated 30 million persons in the United States consider themselves chronic insomniacs. Furthermore, it is estimated that one out of two Americans over the age of 20 suffer from occasional bouts of insomnia. In other countries, both industrial and rural, studies indicate that insomnia occurs with about the same frequency as in the United States. It is quite probable that most estimates and surveys on the incidence of insomnia lean toward the conservative side. It would be hard to find an adult who has never had insomnia, and there is no clear-cut way of determining how many sleepless nights constitute chronic vs. occasional vs. rare insomnia.

One thing seems safe to conclude: wherever there are people, there are insomniacs. But what is insomnia? How do you know if you've got it?

Defining Insomnia for Yourself

You never hear anyone say, "I went to the doctor for a routine checkup and found out I have insomnia. Thank goodness they caught it in time!"

People just don't talk that way about insomnia. There are at least three good reasons why they don't. First of all, insomnia isn't viewed as a life-threatening situation that needs to be "caught in time." Secondly, insomnia isn't something that silently and asymptomatically invades your body without your knowledge. And thirdly, insomnia cannot be diagnosed objectively in a doctor's office or anywhere else. Reliable laboratory tests for insomnia don't exist.

So how do you know if you have insomnia? The answer is: trust your own judgment. Insomnia is not a measurement of how long you sleep or how long it takes you to fall asleep. Nor is it a measurement of certain brain wave patterns that may or may not occur during your sleep. Insomnia is a measurement of how YOU FEEL as a result of your sleep or sleeplessness. Hence, a simple definition: Insomnia is when you don't sleep well and it bothers you.

You more than likely consider yourself an insomniac if: 1) you experience trouble falling asleep, 2) you wake up frequently during the night, 3) you wake up earlier than you desire and can't get back to sleep, or 4) your sleep seems so unsatisfactory that you don't feel well-rested.

Perhaps you have such problems only occasionally. Perhaps you have them frequently. But when you are bothered by these situations—that is, when they affect your waking hours and turn your nighttimes into miniwars against yourself—you are fighting the battle that is called insomnia. No one has to tell you when the battle's on. You know it.

The Lab and the Dilemma of "Objectivity"

Although *you* know when you have insomnia, it would be difficult to get your diagnosis confirmed in a sleep research laboratory. Reliable laboratory tests for insomnia don't exist.

This is not to say that sleep researchers aren't making progress. They are certainly coming up with some valuable information regarding the physiology of sleep. In their laboratories, they can monitor brain activity with EEG (electroencephalograph) machines; they can monitor rapid eye movements (REMS) with EOG (electrooculograph) machines, and they can measure muscular activity with EMG (electromyograph) machines. And they can do all of this while a subject is sleeping in a comfortable laboratory bed. All the subject has to do is wear some painless little electrodes which are pasted on the head and at various places on the body. Contrary to what you might think, the paste and wires do not seem to prevent people from sleeping.

Despite all of this sophisticated equipment, however,

laboratory scientists readily admit that objective criteria do not necessarily make an insomniac. For, as so often happens, what people say about their sleep doesn't always jive with what laboratory studies reveal about their sleep.

For example, a person can insist it usually takes him at least an hour to fall asleep at home; but when he is observed in the lab, his falling-asleep time often proves to be 15 minutes or less. Other insomniacs will insist they haven't slept a wink, when by laboratory standards they have been sleeping for hours. Still others, complaining of chronic insomnia, admit to having slept "like babies" in the confines of the sleep laboratory.

So what's the answer? Do people exaggerate the time it takes them to fall asleep? Perhaps. Do people sleep in a way that somehow doesn't feel like sleep? Perhaps. Are most chronic insomniacs actually suffering from "pseudoinsomnia" or "imaginary insomnia?" Highly unlikely.

The problem with the sleep laboratory is that it's not like home. Not only is the environment different in a laboratory, but many of the external and internal factors that perpetuate insomnia are absent in the laboratory setting. To draw a simple analogy: a person who finds it difficult to relax at home or at work might find it easy to relax while vacationing at a resort. This is not to say that the sleep lab is a resort—but, still, it can offer a kind of temporary respite from the stresses and tensions of everyday living. So it is entirely possible that many people who can't sleep in their own beds would find it easier to sleep in the research laboratory.

What if the sleep scientists could bring their equipment right into a person's home? That still wouldn't solve the problem. For home would no longer be like home in such a situation. It would be like allowing television crews to observe you in your "normal" life. No matter how unobtrusive the crews would be, your "normal" life would have to be altered somewhat.

Thus, no matter how one might try to measure insomnia objectively, it can't be done. What may appear to be a case of "imaginary insomnia" according to objective criteria might actually be a case of "chronic insomnia" on vacation. What may appear to be an exaggerated complaint might be an accurate complaint that just doesn't happen to verify itself in a laboratory setting.

The sleep researcher is faced with a complicated predicament. He cannot seem to measure insomnia objectively. Nor can he determine what kind of a problem it is. Is it a disease? A psychological problem? A physical problem? A habit problem? He's not sure. So he diligently separates subjective insomnia complaints from objective findings in order to search out "the truth." Painstakingly, he looks for all possible electrochemical abnormalities that might turn insomnia into a "real" disease entity. But what if he finds nothing? He can only continue to look for something that may not be there (an "objectively observable abnormality"), while conscientiously disregarding what he knows *is* there (a "subjectively troubled sleeper").

Would it really make any difference if researchers determined that insomnia were an electrochemical abnormality? It is this book's contention that it would not. For, in my estimation, as you learn to reestablish a satisfying sleep pattern, you will at the same time be readjusting any such electrochemical imbalances that may exist.

Would it make any difference if researchers determined that insomnia were a psychological problem? It is this book's contention that it would not. All problems are real, physical imprints on your brain, as you will see in Chapter 5. The real issue is not how to classify insomnia; it's how to get rid of it. In my experience, learning that a problem is "all in your head" in no way enables you to get the problem out of your head. If you continue to believe that what is in your head is imaginary, psychological "nonstuff," you will find it difficult to make a change. For how can you change what isn't there? What is in your head *is* real, physical "stuff"—even if research scientists can't locate the stuff.

There's one other research predicament worth mentioning at this point. That is, sleep research scientists, being unable to describe insomnia objectively, are also at a loss to assess its seriousness objectively. To what extent does insomnia affect productivity? Emotional stability? Disease resistance? Longevity?

In a paper entitled, "Laboratory Studies of Insomnia," Allan Rechtschaffen and Lawrence J. Monroe point out that such questions have not yet been answered adequately. "We really have no good evidence on just how serious insomnia is apart from subjective discomfort," they state. But, as they readily admit, "We do not know the extent of insomnia because we do not know just what it is."[1]

The research problem is a "Catch-22" paradox: How can you define a problem objectively if you can't measure its effects objectively? But how can you measure the effects of a problem objectively if you can't define it objectively?

My guess is that by the time researchers discover something that would be of practical use to you, you will long since have solved your problem.

As for the seriousness of your problem, insomnia in the vast majority of cases is as serious as it feels. Like getting caught in a traffic jam when time is of the essence, insomnia is generally something you dread rather than fear. For, while it doesn't actually threaten your life, it can sure put a damper on it.

No one's insomnia is like anyone else's. The intensity of your problem, the experiences you bring to it, and the factors triggering it are yours and yours alone.

However, there must be something you and all the other insomniacs of the world have in common (besides the fact that you have insomnia). The most obvious thing is your age: virtually all insomniacs are adults. But there is something else you have in common—something all adults are vulnerable to, and you can't see or measure it.

Exit the sleep research laboratories and enter the subjective world of the bedroom. . . .

The Bedroom and the Common Enemy

What goes on when you go to bed and you can't sleep well? Something quite significant goes on. In fact, it's so significant that it constitutes what I call, "the enemy of sleep." Here are some descriptions of sleeping problems from six of my patients. While their complaints are not alike, they are all fighting the same "enemy." From their descriptions, can you tell what the "enemy of sleep" is?

JAN—AGE 36—TEACHER

"I can't fall asleep and it's been like this for about four years . . . ever since I started working with children who had learning disabilities. I guess I became very involved with the children—and I really felt a responsibility to develop effective lesson plans. To this day, I still feel that responsibility. But there are so many difficulties, I can't get the children off my mind. At night when I go to bed, my mind starts racing. I find myself thinking about the problems I'm going to face the next day. Then I start thinking up new lesson plans, and I go on and on for hours. In the beginning, my trouble falling asleep was confined to the weekdays. But now I can't sleep well on the weekends either. It takes me about two hours to fall asleep, and when I wake up I'm so groggy. It takes me another three hours before I start feeling together."

DOROTHY—AGE 62—HOMEMAKER

"I've never had a particularly easy time getting to sleep —I guess I'm kind of a night person. But sleeping became a real problem for me when my husband died two years ago. You see, life without my husband is like a bad dream. There's a bottomless pit of anguish that's always with me. As long as I'm busy with my daily activities, I'm all right. My friends even comment on what a 'pillar of strength' I am. But at night when I get into bed, my facade breaks down. There's nothing between me and that bottomless pit of anguish I feel inside. For the last year or so, I've been taking sleeping pills to keep myself from thinking too much —to stave off the panic. The pills don't always work, though. I hardly ever fall asleep before about 2 A.M., and I'm up by 6 or 7 A.M. As tired as I am, I dread going to bed."

BOB—AGE 46—CORPORATE PRODUCT MANAGER

"I'm losing sleep over my job, and I'll probably lose my job if I don't start getting some sleep. My assistants are all pushing to get to where I am, and my division head watches me like 'Big Brother.' I'm under a lot of pressure to make the right decisions, but so many of my decisions are based on instinct or guesswork. Some of the products I've backed turned out okay—others didn't. I guess I've lost some of my confidence in the last few years. When I go to bed, I start worrying about my job . . . and it progressively gets worse. After a while, as the hours pass me by, I stop worrying about my job and start worrying about how I'll ever get through the day on so little sleep."

LINDA—AGE 30—ARTIST, HOMEMAKER

"I haven't slept well since the baby was born. Billy used to wake up three or four times a night when he was an infant. And for some reason, I was the only one who ever heard him crying. My husband slept right through it all— like a log. Sometimes I even heard Billy before he'd cry: his stirring was enough to wake me up even though his bedroom wasn't that close to ours. Billy is two years old now and rarely gets up in the night. But I still sleep with one ear open—never soundly. I worry and care about my son like all parents do, but I also care about my work and my sleep. Without my sleep, I can't be the kind of artist I want to be, and I can't be the kind of mother I want to be."

STAN—AGE 70—RETIRED POLICEMAN

"I get up too early. A lot of my card-playing buddies have the same problem—and we're all over 65. So maybe it's just a sign of old age. But isn't there anything I can do about it? I get up about 4 A.M., and I can't get back to sleep. I just lie there in bed thinking about things. What else can I do at that hour of the morning? It's hard enough for me to find things to do for the rest of the day. I've had this problem since I retired. And I can tell you this: retirement is not my cup of tea. I do odd jobs whenever I can, but it's not the same as having a place to go every day. I've tried going to bed later so I could get up later—but it doesn't help. When you get up at 4 A.M., you get pretty tired by the time night rolls around. Even when I manage to stay up a few hours later at night, I still get up too early."

GREG—AGE 58—HOSPITAL ADMINISTRATOR

"About a year ago, I was hospitalized for exploratory kidney surgery. Fortunately, the cause of my symptoms turned out to be a benign cyst. But I had a lot of trouble sleeping in the hospital. Who doesn't? When you're thinking about your health, your life, your job, and your family, you can barely close your eyes, let alone sleep. When the nurse would walk in with a sleeping pill for me, I was more than grateful. But when I left the hospital I continued taking sleeping pills at night, and pretty soon I couldn't sleep without them. Of course, this bothered me. It bothered me even more when a few weeks later I found I couldn't sleep with the pills either. Besides my trouble falling asleep, I also have nightmares that wake me up. In this one recurrent nightmare of mine, I'm lying in a hospital bed, and the doctor walks up to me and says he has 'bad news' for me. I wake up in a panic, and it takes me a while to convince myself it was only a dream."

* * *

What goes on in the bedrooms of the world when people can't sleep? What is the "common enemy of sleep?" The answer is THINKING. Not just any kind of thinking. *Excitatory thinking* is what keeps people up. It's the kind of thinking that lights the switches to "ON," turns the volume to "LOUD," and shifts the gears into "AUTOMATIC." It's the kind of agitative thinking you can't seem to control. It just goes ON and On and on . . . involuntarily. Take the six insomniacs just described, for example:

- Jan, the teacher, can't stop thinking about her pupils.
- Dorothy, the 62-year-old widow, reveals that "thinking too much" about her late husband is behind her insomnia problem.
- Bob, the corporate manager, can't stop thinking about his job, his past decisions, his anticipated problems.
- Linda, the mother of Billy, can't get her mind off her responsibilities as a mother and an artist.
- Stan, the retired policeman, thinks excessively about his advancing age, his retirement, and the way it was when he had "a place to go every day."

- Greg, the man who had surgery, can't get his mind off his health and his dependency on drugs.
- All six patients also revealed to me that thinking about sleep had become a problem in itself.

＊ ＊ ＊

When you can't sleep, it's because you're thinking about something that is keeping you up. You can't shift your focus of attention off of some past event, anticipated event, problem, or feeling. Whether it's work, pain, love, money, drugs, sleep, or any other subject that has captured your excitatory thought processes every night, it's your inability to shift your awareness off the subject that makes sleep impossible or difficult: Your wheels just keep spinning, and you can't slow them down.

During your sleepless nights, you undoubtedly know or suspect that you've got to stop thinking about something if you're ever going to get to sleep. You may not be quite sure how something as "mental" as *thinking* could affect something as "physical" as sleeping. But your gut reaction is that this "mental wheel spinning" is what's keeping you up. As a result, perhaps you feel that somehow it's your fault you can't shift your own mind off of whatever it is you're thinking about. Maybe you feel if you used "a little more will power," or "stopped worrying so much," or "stopped taking the pills," you would be able to conquer your insomnia problem.

As you will see in the next chapter, it's no more your fault if you have insomnia than it is the other guy's achievement if he can boast, "Insomnia is one problem I'll never have—I sleep like a log!"

2.

THE OBSOLETE SANDMAN

When I first told Jack L., an insomnia patient, that he could learn to control his own sleep mechanism, he accused me of sounding like his golf pro:

"My golf pro tells me to hold the club firmly but loosely. He tells me to keep my left arm straight but not rigid. He tells me to keep my head down, my hips square, my knees bent—and then to swing naturally! As far as I'm concerned, loose is the opposite of firm; golf is the opposite of natural— and sleep is the opposite of control. You can't possibly fall asleep and be in control at the same time!"

Fortunately, Jack L. did learn how sleep and control could work together for him—and he became quite proficient at self-directing his sleep. Incidentally, as his sleep improved, so did his golf swing. But the point he made about sleep being "the opposite of control" was his way of expressing what I call the "Universal Sandman Myth." As you will see, it is this myth, more than anything else, that makes adults so susceptible to insomnia.

The Universal Sandman Myth

The Universal Sandman Myth states that, "You cannot knowingly and purposely put yourself to sleep. Drugs, boredom, fatigue, music, politicians, alcohol, heavy meals, physiologic occurrences, heavy blows to the skull—almost anything can potentially put you to sleep. But YOU cannot put YOU to sleep."

Because the Universal Sandman Myth is universal, it is found in the words of problem sleepers and never-had-the-problem sleepers:

A Problem Sleeper: "Sometimes when I'm having a bad night, I find myself bargaining with sleep. I say things like, 'Look, Sleep, you've got to sneak up on me when I'm not looking, and just grab me. But you'd better work fast, or I'll see you.' Sleep usually succeeds in grabbing me by about 3 A.M. But it wins by default."

A Never-Had-The-Problem-Sleeper: "I sleep like a baby. All I have to do is close my eyes—and before I know it, ZAP! I'm asleep."

In the preceding descriptions, both individuals are victims of the Sandman Myth. For both view sleep as some-

16

thing that *happens to them.* The "poor sleeper" waits for sleep to "grab" him and the "good sleeper" waits for sleep to "zap" him. Neither has any sense of controlling the actual onset of sleep.

And so it is with most people. We talk about "falling asleep" or being "overcome by sleep," or being "unable to keep our eyes open." We talk about getting ready for bed, climbing into bed, and closing our eyes. But we do not talk about purposely initiating sleep itself. The Universal Sandman Myth says we don't have this capability.

The trouble with the Sandman Myth is that it so often results in drug-resistant, counting-sheep-resistant, knock-down-drag-out insomnia problems. Even those who are lucky enough to get "zapped" to sleep are left vulnerable by the myth: they can just as easily get "zapped" to sleeplessness if some significant event or problem sets their "thinking wheels" spinning. Remember, you too were once lucky enough to get "zapped" to sleep.

The point is: as long as an activity appears to be outside the reaches of one's direct control, as sleep does, one can't do much to prevent the activity from going awry—or staying awry.

Hence, the only way to prevent or conquer insomnia adequately is by taking the whole business of sleeping out of the hands of the sandman and into the realm of your own control. Right now, the idea may strike you as a long shot. The first job of this book, therefore, is to help you reverse the poor odds you've come to expect. For you cannot succeed in directing yourself to sleep when your own expectations are working against you.

The Reality of Expectations

Even if you think you're eligible for a world's record in unsuccessful attempts to conquer insomnia, you must develop a new expectation that you'll succeed this time around. You must begin to expect that the extent of your self-direction can expand. And you must expect that the method described in this book can work for you. In other words, where once you expected failure, you must begin to expect success. This new expectation of success is a *prerequisite* for satisfying, lasting results through the Easy Sleep technique.

But how can you expect something to work if you've never even tried it? It's certainly possible to hope or wish for something to work. But that's not quite the same as *expecting* something to work. In order to expect success, you must have sufficient reason to expect it. I will, therefore, do my best to offer you the practical information you'll need to develop informed, credible, *reasonable expectations* of success through Easy Sleep.

But why are reasonable expectations so vital to your result? Why isn't it enough for this book just to tell you "what to do"? What difference does it make if the method does or doesn't make sense to you? The usual assumption is: "If it works, it works, and if it doesn't, it doesn't."

That "usual assumption" ignores the tremendous physical role expectations play in our lives. An expectation is not an ethereal, psychological flash in the wind, nor is it a subconscious compliance to the "power of suggestion." It is a real, electrochemical recording on your brain. As such, an expectation is as physical as pain or pleasure.

As research has indicated in recent years, everything in your life—everything you see, hear, touch, smell, taste, read, think, say, or do—leaves a trace recording, or IM-PRINT, on your brain. Besides your brain's tremendous recording capacity, it also has a playback capacity. All of your imprints have the capacity to "play back" when re-stimulated. It is this playback, or "memory," capacity that enables you to walk, talk, learn, imagine, analyze, con-template, dream, and perform your daily activities.

Your imprints, therefore, comprise the "programming material" of your brain. In my estimation, the most in-fluential of all this "material" is your expectations. Expecta-tions can signal chemical reactions, hormonal changes, emotional responses, voluntary activities, or involuntary actions. And they can sometimes be more powerful than the most potent of drugs.

As part of your brain's thought system, expectations result from your ability to form conclusions from your observations, experiences, and information. For example, let's say you go on a cruise and get seasick. This experience, like all experiences, is recorded on your brain. The follow-ing year, you go on another cruise, and the same thing happens. After a few such episodes on various boats, you conclude that boating makes you sick. This conclusion is also recorded on your brain, but it's now recorded as an expectation: you *expect* to get sick on boats. If somebody then invites you to go sailing, your expectation imprint plays back, giving you the sense of a plausible, predictable outcome—so you decline the invitation. Now, suppose that instead of going sailing, you go to the movies. And, as luck would have it, the movie is about life aboard a yacht. As you sit in the theater, you find yourself feeling queasy and actually getting seasick! What has happened? Your expectation imprint has been restimulated. Since all imprints are linked by association, the expectation has triggered off the response. There is nothing psychosomatic about the response; it is as real as the way you felt on your first cruise —it is all part of a physical chain of events. Your expectation (a PHYSICAL imprint) signals your response (a PHYSICAL response).

Another example of the "power" of expectations is illustrated in this case history from my internship days:

Mrs. R. suffered from chronic neck pain due to an old injury. Her search for an effective pain medication brought her to the hospital's clinic. She said she had tried numerous pain-relieving medications, including strong narcotics, in the past two years, but none had given her significant relief and most had resulted in considerable nausea and vomiting as side effects. Was there anything else she could take to kill the pain? she asked. Considering that no drugs had helped her in the past and most had caused undesirable side effects, the clinic physician offered Mrs. R. what he called "a strong new pain pill." However, the pill was actually a placebo, which is an inert substance. When Mrs. R. returned to the clinic a few days later, she said the new pills gave her no relief. But, much to my surprise, she also complained that the new pills—the placebos—had caused nausea and vomiting. The clinic staff, of course, decided that Mrs. R.'s problem was "in her head," not her neck, so she was referred to the mental health department.

Although it didn't occur to me at the time, I later came to realize that it was Mrs. R.'s expectations about "pain killers"—her past experiences with other drugs—that had triggered the nausea and vomiting with the placebo. She wasn't "mentally unhealthy" at all.

Every medication, whether it's morphine or a "sugar pill," has a placebo effect. In other words, a person's expectations always come into play when he or she takes a pill. Even in a "double-blind" drug study (when neither the person administering the medication nor the subject receiving the medication knows which pills are the real ones and which are placebos), you cannot distinguish the chemical reactions caused by the pill from the chemical reactions caused by the subject's expectations. The mere act of swallowing a pill carries with it certain expectations, not to mention the additional expectations triggered by the act of participating in an "unbiased" drug study—and certainly also not to mention the expectations triggered when the participant is forewarned that he may be receiving a placebo. Despite all attempts to eliminate bias from drug studies, the fact remains that the only "unbiased" subject is a cadaver.

I hope, therefore, that the early chapters of this book will result in biased readers—readers with reasonable expectations of success through the Easy Sleep technique. For to practice the Easy Sleep method with no reasonable expectation of success would be as futile as trying to relax on an inviting hammock while an overcast sky thunders above you. Working against your expectations can prove to be as frustrating as hitting your head against the wall.

At this point, you have very little reason to expect that these pages will provide the answer to your sleeping problems. But that's understandable considering that this book has been with you for a few minutes or so, whereas the "sandman" has been with you since childhood.

Childhood Expectations

"Everybody's always telling me what to do!" is the child's lament.

Children do not have a strong sense of self-direction. Sometimes they perform activities because other people tell them to. At other times things just seem to happen to them. Even when they're busy doing something on their own, they seldom have a definite sense of why they're doing what they're doing. They may at times feel responsible for something that has happened, but they don't have a clear, purposeful sense of *how* they can make something happen. A child is more a discoverer than a seeker—more curious than deliberate—more deductive than inductive. The child's sense of being-controlled is greater than his sense of self-control.

Children view sleep essentially the same way they view other activities. People tell them to go to sleep; they don't know why they should go to sleep, and have no sense of self-direction regarding sleep. Clearly for the child, sleep is an involuntary activity. It would be difficult to find a child who *wants* to go to sleep except on rare occasions. As far as the child is concerned, the sun sets, the night falls, the call of "Bedtime!" is heard—and the sandman comes to take him off to dreamland. From the setting of the sun to the coming of the sandman, all of these activities are viewed as predictable, expected events, beyond the scope of the child's control and beyond the earshot of his or her wishes.

As children mature their sense of self-direction broadens. By adulthood, they consider and expect rational functioning, voluntary musculature, and, to some extent, emotions, to be within the realm of self-direction or control. Sleep unfortunately falls outside of these areas of *expected control.* At most, the adult feels he can control the time he goes to bed. The time he goes to sleep, however, still remains beyond the scope of his control and beyond the earshot of his wishes.

Thus, as a child you didn't have any expectation that you could self-direct sleep, and as an adult, you still don't. Of course, as a child you didn't need self-direction in order to sleep well. It just happened to you. But then later this thing that had always "just happened" to you somehow "unhappened."

And you are left helpless. The only means you have for deliberately accomplishing anything is through the use of your thinking and reasoning abilities, your muscular coordination, and your capacity to express and explore your emotions. But all of these activities involve being awake, alert, and energetic.

In order to sleep, however, you sense that you must in some way or to some degree stop doing the only things you *can* purposefully do. If you make any attempt to produce sleep deliberately, it seems to elude you. You are thus faced with the peculiar paradox of trying to accomplish something—getting to sleep—by not trying to accomplish anything.

It's easy enough to stop moving your arms and legs. It's not so easy to turn down your emotions, particularly if you can't stop thinking about something. And to deliberately control what you're thinking about is most difficult of all.

Let's say, for example, that thinking about tomorrow's job interview was keeping you up. It would seem quite logical that you would simply get your mind off it and think about something else. After all, everyone says that your mind is your own . . . that you have freedom of thought . . . that you can think about whatever you want to think about. *You are expected to be able to control your thinking.* It thus occurs to you that maybe you just don't want to stop thinking about that job interview badly enough. So you try harder—you exert a little more determination. But the harder you try, the worse it gets. Soon you find yourself thinking about not thinking. And around and around you go. You are stuck.

Changing Your Expectations

Expectations are powerful imprints on your brain—imprints resulting from your ability to form conclusions from your experiences. Since you are always experiencing something new every second of your life, your expectations can and do change.

Take, for example, the functioning of your bowels—one of television advertising's favorite topics. Most individuals expect their bowels to function normally, to "just happen" satisfactorily. But some *significant* situation could disrupt this normal function, resulting in what the TV ads delicately refer to as "irregularity." A few bouts of "irregularity," and a person could certainly change his expectations about "normally" functioning bowels.

An analogous situation would be your expectations regarding sleep. During childhood, you expect sleep to happen to you. Everyone, in fact, expects sleep to happen to him—until some significant event disrupts sleep. Then the expectation starts to change. What you once expected would *simply occur*, you no longer expect will occur.

What about those functions you expect you can *directly* control, as opposed to those functions you expect will "just happen"? Even these expectations can change. For example, a person expects that he can direct himself to walk from one end of the room to another. But suppose a serious accident disrupts this voluntary ability. The person no longer expects to be able to control the movement of his legs to the extent he could in the past.

Again, an analogous example would be your expectations about your thought processes. As an adult, you expect you can control your thoughts. But what if you find yourself in a stressful situation that you can't seem to get off your mind? You reconsider the extent of your control and conclude that you can no longer expect you can control your thoughts to the extent you could in the past.

To sum it all up, this is the way your present expectations regarding sleep evolved:

- As a passive recipient of sleep, you expected sleep to "just happen" to you.

- It stopped happening.
- You have no expectation that you can directly make it happen again. But you *do* expect that if you could control your thinking, your sleep would come.
- You find that you cannot control your thinking.
- You now have no expectation that you can control your thinking, and you have no expectation that you can control your sleeping.

Considering the important role expectations play in the outcome of any therapy, it certainly behooves you to begin changing your present expectations regarding sleep. For, if you are going to attempt to produce sleep willfully and purposefully at your own direction, you will have a far greater chance of success if your expectations complement these purposeful activities.

So, you'll need a new expectation—a new kind of expectation. Your pre-insomnia expectation that sleep would "just happen to you" did not "stick." It was undermined by some experience that disrupted your sleep pattern. Your new expectation, on the other hand, will be the kind that remains firm throughout the inevitable stresses and difficulties we all face from time to time.

Your new expectation will "stick" because it will be a *reasonable* expectation—the opposite of an unreasonable expectation. This, for example, would be an *unreasonable* expectation:

If you follow this book's advice, you will fall asleep the minute your head hits the pillow and will get eight hours of uninterrupted sleep every single night for the rest of your life.

A *reasonable* expectation, in contrast, would sound something like this:

If you understand and practice the principles of Easy Sleep, you will be able to obtain satisfactory sleep, although on some nights it may take you more time to get to sleep than on others. After all, occasional tensions and problems are an inescapable part of life, and we all take our problems to bed sometimes.

With the Easy Sleep approach, you still may face an occasional sleeping problem. But it will be about as troublesome to you as a minor stub of the toe. That is, it may delay you briefly, but it will not prevent you from directing yourself to where you want to go.

* * *

As I stated before, the first job of this book is to help you reverse the poor sleeping odds you've come to expect. By recognizing the tangibility of your expectations—their existence as electrochemical brain imprints capable of signaling real, physical reactions—you are already tipping the odds in your favor. For you now understand the necessity for changing your present expectations and developing new, reasonable expectations that you can direct yourself to sleep. By the time you're ready to practice the Easy Sleep concentration technique, you will have every reason to expect that it will work.

In the next chapter, you will see why many of the sleep remedies you may have tried did not work. You will see how all those well-intentioned "sleep panaceas" are really "adult dosage" varieties of that old, exhausted sandman.

3.

THOSE ELUSIVE SLEEP PANACEAS

If you're thirsty, you look for something to drink. If you're cold, you look for something to warm you up. And if you are bothered by sleeplessness, you look for something to help you sleep.

The awareness of discomfort always begets the search for relief. But the problem is: what you seek is not necessarily what you find, and what you would like to happen is not necessarily what ends up happening. More often than not, relief from insomnia continually eludes you.

All of which makes insomnia a big business. Americans spend about $500 million a year for prescription medications to help them sleep. Added to this are the hundreds of millions of dollars spent on nonprescription medications, electronic devices such as sound emitters, vibrators, and head warmers, special beds and pillows, alcoholic beverages, courses in yoga, meditation and self-hypnosis, numerous visits to family doctors and psychiatrists, earplugs, eye masks, and countless other sleeping aids. In total, it's almost impossible to measure the amount we spend in our search for that good night's sleep. There are, in fact, so many different remedies and aids available to the insomniac that it would be far too time consuming to add them all up. While at the library one day, I pulled out three reference books and within 10 minutes found 807 different sleep remedies.

It is easy enough to understand why this plethora of sleeping aids and agents exists. Remember, the Universal Sandman Myth (Chapter 2) states: *"Almost anything* can potentially put you to sleep. But YOU cannot put YOU to sleep."* If you have no expectation that you can do much YOURSELF to regain your sleeping ability, you have no choice but to look outside of yourself for an answer. And *"almost anything"* covers a lot of territory. With territory that broad, you have plenty to choose from.

But you also have plenty of opportunities to fail. After a number of unsuccessful attempts to regain your sleeping ability through one means or another, you begin to expect failure. You can easily get the feeling, "I've tried everything, and nothing works."

By understanding something about those sleep remedies that didn't work to your satisfaction, you will find it easier to replace your old expectation of failure with a new expectation of success this time around.

So let's take a look at those remedies. For purposes of

simplicity, I have divided the various sleep remedies you may have tried into five general categories.

The Sleeping Pill Panacea

Barbiturates, tranquilizers, muscle relaxers, over-the-counter remedies: millions of people swallow billions of pills to get to sleep. When effective, the pills seem to turn off your excitatory thinking, calm you down, lull you to sleep—perhaps, even "knock you out." So what's wrong with sleeping pills?

I am sure you're already familiar with the potential dangers, contraindications, and adverse effects associated with various drugs. But to state that one pill is safer than another or one pill is stronger than another would really be an exercise in speculation. For, as you saw in the last chapter, it is quite impossible to separate the chemical effects caused by a medication from the chemical effects caused by the expectations and sensitivity of the person taking it. If a sleeping pill is making you feel worse instead of better, then the pill is wrong for you. Right now the issue is YOU, not statistical findings or drug abuse potentials.

If taking a sleeping pill every night were the answer for you, you wouldn't be reading this book. If taking an occasional sleeping pill solved your problem, you wouldn't be reading this book. The relevant question here is: Do sleeping pills work for you? My guess is that you would either answer, "No," or "Sometimes," or "They used to."

The most common shortcoming associated with sleeping medications is that people tend to develop tolerance to them quite quickly. The usual explanation for this tolerance factor is that your body builds up a resistance to the chemical properties of various drugs at particular dosage levels. In other words, your body has a protective mechanism which adjusts to certain toxins, so they no longer have an adverse effect on your system. According to this theory, it thus becomes necessary to increase the dosage of certain drugs in order to produce the results you desire. Apparently, what your body desires and what you desire are at odds with one another.

This widely accepted theory of tolerance, which undoubtedly has some truth to it, once again minimizes the role of the individual who's swallowing the pill. It's as if *you* and *your body* were somehow two separate entities— as if what you want, think, or feel has nothing whatsoever to do with what happens within your body. It's simply not so.

While you may have frequent sleeping problems, the intensity of your problem varies from night to night. The intensity of a sleeping pill, however, remains the same. So, it's not necessarily a question of the pill's action weakening, but rather of your sleeping problem intensifying. Added to this is your expectation that tolerance will develop—an expectation that makes you worry about what you will do next: "Should I take more?" "Should I change medications?" "Should I give up pills altogether?" "What if I can't?" "What if I become an addict?" "Maybe I'm already an addict." You may also worry about the mere fact that you "need" a pill in the first place. As your worries mount, your insomnia mounts, and your problem becomes too big for the pill. You may even find yourself in the "Thinking-About-Pills-Is-Keeping-Me-Up" trap. All of these factors come into play when you swallow a pill. All of these factors contribute to your reaction to a pill. It's not just the .5 gm. of this or the 10 mg. of that which dictates the results.

It has been suggested by some researchers that sleeping pills *cause* chronic insomnia. The theory here is that certain drugs cause disturbed sleep, tolerance, and withdrawal effects all in one handy little formulation. Thus, a person takes a drug; his sleep becomes disturbed; he attempts to stop taking the drug; his sleep is even more disturbed (a withdrawal effect); he then takes more drugs; he becomes a so-called, "drug-dependent insomniac."

While it's true that many insomniacs are drug-dependent, I believe it would be misleading to conclude that the pills *cause* the insomnia. Drug problems can certainly serve to reinforce or intensify sleep problems. But, in my opinion, they are not to blame for causing them. If a person were dependent on drugs for the relief of chronic pain, would one conclude that the drugs *caused* the pain?

Sometimes drugs are both useful and effective. At other times drugs become so closely associated with a problem that they actually become a trigger for perpetuating the problem. But they are just one of a million such triggers, as you will see in Chapter 5.

Drugs alone cannot be credited for causing a problem or curing a problem. The few chemical activities caused by a pill cannot possibly compete with the millions of chemical activities produced by your brain.

(Note: If you are now taking regular or heavy doses of

any sleeping medication, be sure that any attempts at withdrawal be carried out gradually and under the supervision of your doctor. A program of gradual drug withdrawal combined with the regular practice of the Easy Sleep technique is recommended to help you reestablish a satisfying sleep pattern with minimal difficulty.)

The Dull-Book Panacea

Included in this classification of sleeping aids are the familiar what-to-do suggestions that hardly anybody can stand doing. These include: reading a dull book; counting sheep; engaging in mild, unstressful, non-competitive exercise daily; avoiding cigarettes and alcohol in excess of two drinks daily; avoiding coffee, tea, cola drinks, and all beverages containing caffeine; avoiding all "mentally stimulating" discussions, books, movies, and games before retiring.

The idea behind these suggestions is that boredom puts people to sleep, and stimulation keeps them awake. What few proponents of some of these suggestions realize, however, is that writing off coffee, cigarettes, and other "bad habits" can be extremely stressful. Trying to stop doing all those things that are "bad for you" is supposed to help you relax. But the effort involved can be far from relaxing and sleep inducing.

What about engaging in pre-bedtime *boring* activities? Even if you could read dull books and participate in dull activities on a nightly basis, you would probably run into the tolerance problem again. Then you would have to read two dull books instead of one, count 200 sheep instead of 100, etc. . . . you might even become bored to tears, which is worse than insomnia.

The Warm Milk Panacea

Drink a glass of warm milk, eat a high-protein bedtime snack, take a warm bath. These are among the "natural sedative" remedies. Milk, for example, contains an amino acid called tryptophan which, according to laboratory tests, appears to have a mild sedative effect.

The mild sedative effects of foods, drinks, and warm baths may well have a scientific validity. The mild sedative effects of water beds, massages, and machines that simulate the sound of rain may also have a scientific validity. But sleeping pills also have a scientific validity: There is certainly enough evidence to support their sleep-producing chemical properties. The problem, however, is that the chemical effects produced by your expectations can be far stronger than the chemical effects produced by foods, drugs, and warm liquids, whether of the bathing, drinking, or sleeping-on variety. Also, once again, the tolerance factor must be considered. A glass of warm milk may get you to sleep one night. But the next night you may need the milk and the bath, and the next night you may need the milk and the snack and the bath, and the next night you may even try chomping on a grilled cheese sandwich while bathing in a tub of warm milk. The search for the "natural low" can be about as fruitless as the search for the "natural high" or the search for the perfect drug.

The Reassurance Panacea

Many doctors and sleep experts advocate "reassurance" as the best and safest method for treating common insomnia complaints. The underlying rationale for this approach is that many insomniacs are actually "perfectly healthy" people who simply worry too much about their sleep. While there may be some superficial validity in the rationale, the method of treatment that follows is often grossly inadequate. Here, for instance, are common examples of treatment-by-reassurance. In each example, the doctor is speaking to the patient:

"You're probably getting a lot more sleep than you imagine, so stop worrying about it."

"The reason you get up at 4 A.M. is because you simply don't need as much sleep as you used to. You're perfectly normal."

"When you get in bed, don't think about what you're going to do the next day."

"Relax more. Don't be afraid to let go. Think pleasant thoughts."

"Stop wanting to go to sleep. Talk yourself out of your need for sleep. Use a little reverse psychology on yourself."

The problem with all of these well-meaning words of encouragement is that no one tells you *how* to stop worrying or *how* to relax or *how* to believe your own reverse psychology. If an insomniac could stop worrying, etc., he undoubtedly would.

Also included in the reassurance category are words of

advice such as: 1) Don't go to bed until you're sleepy; 2) If you can't fall asleep, get out of bed and do something; 3) Go to bed at the same time every night; 4) Establish pre-sleep rituals and follow your routine every night.

Obviously, suggestions 1 and 3 contradict each other. But beyond that, the suggestions are largely irrelevant. In the first place, a lot of insomniacs are sleepy, but they just can't sleep. In the second place, getting out of bed does not solve the problem of what to do when you get back in bed. In the third place, going to bed at the same time is easy enough—the difficulty is in going to sleep. And finally, pre-sleep rituals (e.g., checking the locks on all the doors, brushing your teeth, opening the window two inches, getting in bed from the left side, etc.) can sometimes distract you from your sleep problems. Most people *can* manage to think and brush their teeth at the same time. Becoming a compulsive slave to rituals, furthermore, can make sleeping more difficult: once you finally get between the sheets, it's easy to fall into the trap of wondering if you have forgotten to do something . . . and out of bed you go to recheck the doors, windows, etc. Thus, problems are added to problems.

The "Mind" Panacea

Meditation, self-hypnosis, yoga, and Zen are exercises designed to help you achieve an "altered state of consciousness." They have all been used with varying degrees of success in treating insomnia. But there are problems here, too.

One of the biggest problems with the so-called mind-control techniques is that they depend on your predisposition toward them. Many people, for example, consider meditative exercises to be activities reserved for mystics, disciples, believers. As one woman put it, "I'm not looking for a religious experience. I'm looking for sleep." Others maintain that they are simply not hypnotizable, not suggestible. Still others state that they "don't have the patience" to concentrate on a "mantra" or a word or an object for 20 or 40 minutes. For one reason or another, a lot of people consider the idea of "achieving an altered state of consciousness" to be just a bit "too far out."

Another problem with meditative techniques is they demand that you maintain a passive attitude as you practice them—an attitude of *letting something happen*, as opposed to *making something happen*. Exactly what you're supposed to "let happen" is never really defined, so it's hard to know if you're "getting it" or not. Furthermore, as a passive recipient of the meditative experience, you may get to sleep, and you may not. But, if you don't get to sleep, there's nothing you can do about it: you can't be passive and active at the same time. It becomes largely a hit-or-miss proposition.

Various techniques such as biofeedback and progressive relaxation have many of the same drawbacks as the meditative disciplines. Although they do not have mystical connotations, these techniques do have their shortcomings.

Progressive relaxation is a technique for relaxing your voluntary musculature so that you can achieve a deep state of relaxation. Biofeedback is an electronic offshoot of "visceral learning." Through concentration on auditory or visual signals, you are supposed to be able to elicit the state of relaxation you desire.

Both biofeedback and progressive relaxation require that their subjects maintain passive attitudes—that they *not try*. By concentrating on "beeps" or muscle groups, the desired state of relaxation is supposed to happen. Unfortunately, it doesn't always happen. And when it doesn't, it just doesn't. Since you are warned not to analyze your failures nor deliberately try to change something you're doing, all you can do is wait. And waiting is what you're already doing when you get in bed at night.

On the other hand, if you do manage to achieve a state of deep relaxation through these techniques, there is no assurance that sleep will follow. Sleep may be a beneficial side-effect of relaxation, but if sleep doesn't follow, what can you do? You can't willfully produce a side-effect. Side-effects are unintended results.

Problem #1: The Passive Factor

Whether it's a pill, a glass of milk, a dull book, a few words of encouragement, or 20 minutes in the lotus position that promise to bring sleep to you, all such remedies have obvious shortcomings. One shortcoming is that they put you in the position of being a passive recipient of their benefits. You simply have no sense of control over the outcome. All you can do is sit back and hope for the best.

Perhaps you can think up rational explanations for why these remedies work when they work and why they fail when they fail. But you have no way of applying your rea-

soning to make the remedies work. At most, you can conclude, "I understand why this is supposed to work, but it
just doesn't work for me."

In other words, all your thinking and reasoning abilities
just don't do you a bit of good when you are given instructions such as, "Let it happen," or "Swallow this and wait,"
or "Don't worry, sleep will come." Taken altogether, such
instructions really translate as, "The sandman will return."
Of course, that's kind of hard to believe when night after
night the sandman skips over you.

Any passive approach to problem-solving is inherently
hit-or-miss. When there is no self-direction, there is no self-
assurance. There is only luck—and how many of us are
consistently lucky?

Problem #2: The Tolerance Factor

The second major shortcoming of most sleep remedies
is that they all attempt to do something *to* you, but they
haven't any idea of who YOU are. In their attempts to
break down your resistance to sleep, they fail to recognize
the strong stuff you're made of. They try to overpower you,
but you are the one who unwittingly overpowers them.
For you are the one with the "tolerance factor"—tolerance
is part of you, not the remedies themselves.

Tolerance is usually spoken of in relation to drugs and
environmental toxins. Your body, it is said, adjusts to various chemical "insults" which could potentially threaten
your physiologic equilibrium. There is certainly no doubt
that you have various immunological and resistance mechanisms that enable you to tolerate environmental toxins,

viruses, and bacterial invasions. But that kind of resistance, when it's running well, is carried on by the autonomic areas of your brain. You are not aware of fighting off every virus you come in contact with, nor do you need to be.

When it comes to sleeping pills, tolerance is quite another phenomenon. Swallowing a pill is a deliberate action. All your awareness is focused on the activity. All your expectations about what will happen are triggering off numerous electrochemical responses. Tolerance to sleeping pills is not purely an immunological survival mechanism: It is also an expectation mechanism—an expectation that any good results you get are likely to be temporary. And as is so often the case, expectations end up being self-fulfilling prophecies.

Just as you can become tolerant to sleeping pill remedies, you can become tolerant to almost any insomnia panacea. A warm bath, a run around the block, sitting in a chair for 20 minutes twice a day and silently repeating "Om, Om, Om, Om. . . ." All can trigger off tolerance reactions. The basic difference between tolerance to pills and tolerance to these other remedies is that you tend to discard the non-pill remedies when they stop working. Because of your expectations about pills, however, you tend to search for a stronger medication or to increase your dosage.

Whenever you are aware of a problem and you seek to relieve it, your expectations come into play. Any of the sleep panaceas can result in so-called tolerance, as they fail to meet the growing intensity of your problem. Combine the growing intensity of your problem with the growing intensity of your expectations of failure and you end up with an overpowering tolerance to any external sopo-rific formula.

The Central Remedy

While other sleep remedies attempt to overpower your problem, this book's remedy is devised to solve it. A sprained ankle can only be healed centrally—by your own healing mechanisms. The same is true of insomnia.

A central cure for insomnia is a cure accomplished by you, deliberately. It is a self-directed cure. It is going right to where the problem is, and changing it.

Where is the problem? It's in your brain.

What is the problem? It's an imprint, a "Can't Sleep" imprint.

What will you change? You will change the "Can't Sleep" imprint to a "Can Sleep" imprint. You will also change the activities and expectations associated with these imprints.

Because you will be the one in charge of your own sleep, you will not run into tolerance. If one night is a bit more tense for you than another, you will be able to adjust the technique to fit your own needs at the time.

In order to direct yourself to sleep, you will need to understand something about the mechanism of sleep. For it would be difficult to direct something without knowing what it is you're directing. What is sleep? And what is going on in that extraordinary powerhouse called your brain? The next chapter will unlock the mystery.

4.

A PRACTICAL, UNMYSTERIOUS VIEW OF SLEEP

Sleep ... the big mystery. It's a reputation that began thousands of years ago and continues to live on. Philosophers ponder it, poets muse about it, and scientific investigators work at unraveling it. In the "we-still-don't-have-the-answers-to-it" category, sleep has managed to hold its own.

Unlocking the mystery of sleep has so captured the imagination of scientists that sleep research has become a specialty unto itself. Working all night long and sometimes around the clock, sleep researchers observe and gather data that might give clues as to the real nature of sleep. For 25 years, since the first modern sleep laboratory was developed, the data have accumulated. But the researchers have not yet found the key. They have still to discover to their own satisfaction what sleep means or what purpose it serves. They acknowledge the common-sense answers to the riddles of sleep, but neither common sense nor theory counts as fact from the scientist's point of view.

Is it necessary to await all the facts before you can get the kind of sleep you want? In my estimation, it's neither necessary nor practical. Perhaps someday the insomniac will find it useful to understand the precise metabolic roles serotonin, dopamine, and norepinephrine play in the sleep process. Perhaps someday an exact understanding of REM (rapid eye movement) and NREM (non-REM) sleep will be of some practical value to the insomniac. But, as William C. Dement, a noted authority on sleep from Stanford University, has stated, "... (A) researcher is obliged to state the facts—to describe phenomena in terms of what we know. Speaking in such a strict manner with regard to REM sleep, I can only say: 'It's there. It looks the way I've described it.' We just don't know yet, despite twenty years of intensive research, why it's there. In many ways, REM periods resemble epileptic seizures. Perhaps they are equally as useful."[1]

What it really boils down to is that waiting for the "facts" could prove to be a colossal waste of time. The "facts" might end up having no meaning or practical application whatsoever. If you had to wait to investigate all the different electrochemical facts that would enable you to move your hand, you'd never get around to moving your hand. You don't need all that information to move your hand. And you don't need all that information in order to direct yourself to sleep.

But what do you need to know about sleep in order to turn it on? You need to know what the activity is that you're turning on, and what the activity is that you're turning off. What I now offer you is a common-sense, theoretical view of sleep; that is, an understanding of sleep that will have a practical application for you. Since my purpose here is to give you information you can use—not to give you an anatomy lesson—I will avoid the use of scientific terminology and anatomical detail. The general concepts I'll describe are, however, based on neurophysiologic information, research and practical experience.

Brain Energy—The Stuff You Run On

If anyone ever tells you that your problems are all in your head, you can respond with assurance, "Of course they are. If I didn't have my head, I wouldn't have any problems ever!"

Within your head is the powerhouse of all your life's activities—the *central control area.* It is your brain. Your brain integrates everything from your heartbeats to your thoughts and feelings. Your brain is the powerhouse; your brain energy is the power.

Brain energy. It is a force as real as the power that comes from an electrical socket. It is, in fact, the determinant of life. For hundreds of years it was believed that life was determined by the presence of a heartbeat or a pulse. But in recent years—as recently as 1974—science has discovered that life can more accurately be measured in brainwave terms. The presence of brain waves on an EEG indicates real, tangible electrochemical activity going on in the brain. Brain energy is the stuff you run on. It's the stuff that makes all systems go.

What does brain energy do? First of all, it turns signals into imprints. As was stated in Chapter 2, every stimulation you receive—everything you hear, see, smell, feel, say, or do—is recorded on your brain as an imprint. But, in order to get recorded in the cortical or "storage" area of your brain, a signal must first receive some energy. It must pass through your brain's "energy power pack area." This power pack area, comprising what is known as the reticular formation and limbic system, amplifies the incoming signals so that recordings can be made.

All of these recordings in your brain—these imprints—are linked by association to other imprints. For example, the visual imprint of a red traffic light and the word imprint of "stop" are linked by association in your brain.

Besides turning signals into imprints, your brain energy also facilitates the playback of associated imprints. The red light imprint and the "stop" imprint have the capacity to feed back into the energy power pack area, giving you the ability to react, the energy to actually stop.

Without the power pack area of your brain, you would be incapable of picking up signals or stimulations. Without the recording and playback capacity of your brain, the signals you receive would have no meaning, no function. So, putting it all together, what you have working for you is a brain energy system that enables you to be truly human; to have a tremendous capacity to learn, feel, and do many things.

And it *is* all in your head. It's an energy system that is in constant motion as it picks up messages and sends out messages. It is an energy system that is constantly amplifying, recording, and modifying, building experience onto experience in a highly complex yet wonderfully organized manner. There is no computer on earth that can handle the amount of data your brain handles, filing millions of bits of information and producing millions of readouts a day. And there is no computer on earth that can program itself *with a sense of self.* Only your brain can do all that.

"YOU"—*The Biggest Imprint*

The energy power pack area of your brain is actually a highly complex circuitry network consisting of numerous systems, regions, and subdivisions. But, for simplicity, I will divide the power pack into three general areas. The *behavioral* power pack area contains the energy circuits used for verbal communication, thinking, reasoning, moving your muscles, performing all those activities we usually think of as "voluntary." The *emotional* power pack area contains the energy circuits used to impart feelings or tones to experiences. The *autonomic* area consists of the circuitry used for running internal organs, hormonal functions, and all those activities generally considered "involuntary." As you will see in the next chapter, the words "voluntary" and "involuntary" are artificial distinctions implying a separateness that is not quite that absolute.

Although I have separated the brain's power pack into three energy areas, I should mention that all the areas are interconnected and associated with one another. Obviously, for example, a "behavioral" game of racquetball can affect the "autonomic" production of sweat. Similarly, an "emotional" feeling of anxiety can affect the "behavioral" act of delivering a speech. And an "autonomic" bout with the flu can affect the "emotional" feeling of fitness. The interconnections between the behavioral, emotional, and autonomic areas are always at work to some extent. For the purposes of this book, however, the emphasis will be on the area I'll call "behavioral." It is this area that supplies us with the practical information about sleep, its meaning, its purpose, its functioning, and its occasional malfunctioning.

The behavioral energy circuit system comprises the highest nervous system energy use. It's the hottest, busiest, most complex energy circuitry in your brain.

What makes it so hot? YOU do. In your daily life, your *sense of self* (your awareness, your consciousness) is largely occupied in the performance of behavioral activities. When you speak of wanting certain things, thinking certain things, doing certain things, you are primarily referring to your use of behavioral energy. Intricately tied with this energy use is your sense of purpose, sense of awareness, sense of self. To sum it up, most of the time you know what you're doing. You have a sense of knowing where you are.

What is a sense of knowing, a sense of involvement, a sense of one's self? To begin with, the sense of self is an imprint. It is the "biggest" and most intense imprint on your brain. When played back into the energy pool (the power pack area), this imprint gives you a sense of orientation to person, place, time, how you're feeling, what you're doing, and what's being done to you. Therefore, I will call this imprint your *self-anchoring imprint,* or your *self-awareness imprint.*

In 1916, the Nobel prize-winning physiologist Ivan Petrovich Pavlov stated that one of the strongest reflexes accompanying human and animal life was the "orienting or focusing" reflex. This reflex, he said, was exhibited by animals and humans in their daily endeavors "to grasp or test every new phenomenon or object with the appropriate receptor surfaces, the corresponding sense organs."[2]

In light of recent neurophysiologic information, we can now view Pavlov's "orienting reflex" as an actual brain recording or imprint* Neurosurgery has revealed time and again that it is possible to evoke the "reliving" of long-forgotten experiences in a patient by electrical stimulation of certain cortical areas of the brain.

So, from Pavlov's theory as to the existence of an orienting reflex, we can now add recent scientific findings and conclude that an *orienting* or *self-anchoring imprint* exists in the cortex of your brain.

As you go through your daily life, this intense self-anchoring imprint is in constant use. Furthermore, the imprints that are linked to it number in the billions. Your name, your background, your sex, your appearance, your talents, your occupation, and your opinions are a mere fraction of the vast number of imprints associated with your self-anchoring imprint, or your sense of self. Taken together, all these imprints add up to your concept of YOU.

---

* Throughout this book, when I use the term "imprint," it will be in the singular. However, this is just to simplify matters, for any message recorded on the brain actually consists of thousands of bits of recorded information.

When you talk about your ability to communicate, your desire to solve a problem, your motivation, your achievements, your failures, your goals, your responsibilities, and your ability to think, form abstractions and be creative, you are talking about the most complex and most important uses of your brain's energy. These behavioral energy circuits are thus the busiest and hottest.

Since your behavioral circuits are primarily consumed by your self-awareness, or self-anchoring, activities, I will refer to the largest portion of the behavioral energy power pack as the *self-awareness energy circuitry*. It is this circuitry, working in conjunction with your self-anchoring imprint, that allows you to do all the things you do with an accompanying sense of yourself as a person—a sense of your connection to what's going on around and within you.

Being Awake

Since being awake and being asleep are the most obvious natural states of the living human brain, it seems that an understanding of one could unlock the mystery of the other. And it does.

Very simply put: Being awake is being AWARE of yourself, relatively speaking.

In the awake state, your self-anchoring imprint is in high gear. Your awareness energy circuits are in an electrically active state. Whether your awareness is primarily focused on incoming signals (for example, the ringing of your telephone) or past recorded imprints (such as reflecting on yesterday's phone conversation) you maintain that "sense of self" when you are awake. In other words, when you're awake, you have a sense of connection between yourself and what's happening around you.

In the awake state there are, naturally, shades of awareness. When conversing with a friend, for example, you may be more aware of yourself and your surroundings than you would be if you were sitting back in a relaxing chair and listening to music. But such degrees of awareness are understandable, considering you're never *exactly* the same from one minute to the next. You are always using either more or less energy than you were an instant before.

Being awake, therefore, is when your sense of self—your orientation, your consciousness, your self-awareness—is playing and replaying at a relatively high frequency.

In summary, there are various ways of describing what it means to be awake:

- It's being aware of yourself in relationship to your environment.
- It's when your self-anchoring imprint is in high gear.
- It's when your sense of self, or orientation, is playing and replaying with relative intensity.
- It's when you are using a proportionately large amount of energy from your behavioral power pack area (your self-awareness circuitry)—the area associated with deliberate activity, problem solving, goal seeking, communicating, judging, thinking, reflecting, knowing, and doing.

There is one more point that should be made about the awake/aware state. Having an awareness of what you're doing or experiencing does not necessarily mean having control over what you're doing or experiencing. Although a good portion of your self-awareness energy circuitry is occupied in the performance of deliberate, voluntary activity, you can also be aware of nondeliberate, involuntary activity. Hence, your awareness circuits, which are in high gear as you run to catch a bus (a deliberate activity), are also in high gear when you are conscious of a muscle twitch or a feeling of nervous tension (non-deliberate activities).

It is not *what you are aware of* that constitutes being awake: it's the fact *that you are actively aware* that constitutes being awake.

Being Asleep

Sleep is more or less the converse of being awake. If being awake is when your self-anchoring imprint is in high gear, being asleep is when your self-anchoring imprint is in low gear. When you're awake, your sense of self—your self-awareness energy circuits—are playing at a relatively high frequency. When you're sleeping, your self-awareness energy circuits are playing at a relatively low frequency.

Thus we arrive at a definition of sleep: Sleep is the relative inhibition of your self-anchoring imprint.[3] The reason I have used the qualifier "relative" is because there is never a time when you are *totally* unaware, provided your brain is functioning within the realm of "normal." Your self-anchoring imprint is always playing back to some degree, unless you are unconscious, comatose, or dead.

Since you can be sure you are none of the above, you can safely conclude that you are never *completely* unaware. Even when your self-anchoring imprint is in low gear, it still has life and energy. So, although your sense of self is certainly minimal during sleep, you are still capable of responding to sounds and events around you. You are capable of being aroused in the event of an emergency such as a fire alarm or a shout for help. You are also capable of being aroused in the event of a pleasant invitation such as a touch or a whisper.

Sleep is, without a doubt, an immense reduction in your use of awareness energy; you are relatively unconnected to your environment. But your awareness is not dead. It's just turned down to a low frequency. During certain stages of sleep your awareness is lower than it is during other stages, but it always has the capacity to turn higher if the need should arise.

What Sleep Is For

Every waking and sleeping moment of your life is consumed with amplifying, recording, and modifying external and internal signals. Your brain's energy system is always active. The only *significant* difference between wakefulness and sleep is that when you're awake, your self-awareness energy circuitry is in high gear; when you're asleep, these circuits are relatively inhibited.

The logical question is: What's this gearshifting for? What's the purpose of sleep?

It's a two-part answer. Part One: Sleep is necessary to "cool off" those hot awareness energy circuits in your brain —the circuits associated with your sense of self. Part Two: Sleep is necessary for "cleaning up" the imprint storage area of your brain.

Cooling Off

Why do your awareness energy circuits need to cool off? For the same reason that all of your energy circuits need cooling-off time. Your body cannot continue to perform any of its functions efficiently without having some rest periods. If you raise your arm, eventually you have to lower it; if you stare at something, eventually you have to blink; if you're jogging, eventually you have to rest; if your heart is "pounding," eventually it will need to slow up. Resting is our means for getting our energy back.

With the exception of your awareness activities, all of your other functionings can probably get sufficient rest relatively quickly and effortlessly. Your internal organs, for example, go through periods of high activity and low activity throughout the day and night. Furthermore, it seems reasonable to conclude that many of these non-awareness activities don't require such intensive rest because they don't tax your energy systems to the degree your awareness activities do.

Your awareness (orientation, conscious) activities can only get their rest by becoming inhibited. And because they require so much energy to function well, they require a more intense and lengthy inhibition than other activities do. While it's true that you can "rest your mind" to some degree by relaxing, meditating, or taking some sort of pleasure break, apparently such "time outs" are not sufficient to do the necessary cooling-off job. Until such time as someone can come up with an alternative, sleep will remain the most efficient way of obtaining the degree of rest and rejuvenation required by your highest nervous system activities.

Your awareness energy circuits must cool off if they are to continue to provide the power necessary for getting through your daily life satisfactorily. When they don't cool off sufficiently, you can actually feel it. The feeling is so common that millions of people express it daily when they say things like, "I don't have any energy"; "I'm a little slow today"; "I've just been dragging around all day." All of these statements are reflections of an awareness energy system that is overworked and underrested—a system in need of cooling off, recharging.

Cleaning Up

The cleaning-up role of sleep is as important to your daily functioning as the cooling-off role. Every day your brain records millions of new stimulations which are associated with your sense of self. Your self-anchoring imprint is constantly being used, renewed, and reinforced every single second of your waking life.

Although all these new signals are instantly linked to past recorded imprints and are quickly "filed" in the storage area of your brain, further "linking and filing" is essential to proficient functioning.

This additional linking and filing—the clean-up process —can only be done efficiently while you are sleeping. With your self-awareness relatively inhibited, your brain has the chance to run its newest imprints back through your energy power pack without much interference from YOU. If your awareness were not inhibited, you would probably impede the clean-up process in two ways: 1) You would be occupying so much of the energy circuitry with your awareness activities, there wouldn't be much energy available for cleanup; 2) You would react in a positive way to the imprints as they ran through your energy circuitry during cleanup—you would experience the imprints as if they were *actually* happening—in a word, you would be hallucinating. Fortunately, because your self-awareness is relatively inhibited during sleep, you experience the clean-up process as a dream, if you're aware of experiencing it at all.

Sleep facilitates effective cleanup. And cleanup is necessary for putting things into perspective—for putting the memory bank in order. During sleep, as your brain runs through its newest imprints, many older imprints follow along in a procession—an association procession. It's kind of like the word game children sometimes play, where one says a word and the others build upon it to see what they come out with. One youngster starts off by saying "baseball," for example. The next one says "bat." The next says "stick." And on it goes from "stick" to "stone" to "rock" to "sand" to "beach" to "water" to "wet" to "my baby brother's diapers," which is followed by so much giggling that the game is deemed a success.

As your imprints proceed through your energy areas during sleep, they intricately connect themselves to other past experiences or imprints. In the process they sort themselves out. Some imprints take a position in the "front" of the memory files, and others are moved further toward the back of the files. In general, the imprints that received a large amount of awareness energy when you were awake, such as finding the solution to a problem that had been plaguing you for weeks, tend to be filed close to the "front." The imprints that occupied little of your awareness energy when you were awake, such as the color of someone's tie, get filed in the "back," depending on the tie, of course— there are some you never forget!

Essentially, the clean-up process is your brain's way of efficiently integrating the new information with the old. It's a reorganization, systemization process that allows today's experiences to become tomorrow's memories, today's thoughts to become tomorrow's knowledge, and today's input to become tomorrow's reference material.

In everyday language, the benefits of sleep's clean-up process may be found in statements such as: "Time heals all wounds"; "You'll feel better in the morning"; "Everything looks better in the light of day"; "Go home, sleep on it, and give me your answer tomorrow."

Feeling With-It

After your brain's energy circuitry has "cooled off" and your imprint filing system has "cleaned up," you are recharged and ready for the next day.

Hence, the purpose of sleep could be summed up in the expression: "Feeling with it." In other words, efficient sleep helps you to feel alert, attentive, and "tuned in" as you go about the business and pleasures of daily living.

Looking briefly at results of laboratory sleep deprivation experiments, it becomes quite clear that the fundamental role of sleep is to provide individuals with this "with-it" factor. Time and again, research studies have indicated that prolonged sleep deprivation primarily affects an individual's concentration, his mood, and his speed in performing various tasks. Although this "decreased mental agility" varies from individual to individual, and although a good night's sleep quickly restores whatever impairments may have resulted from the sleep loss, most researchers will agree that total sleep deprivation chiefly affects cognitive processes and subjective feelings of well-being.

The differences between voluntary sleeplessness in the laboratory setting and involuntary insomnia in the home setting are numerous. The most obvious difference is that laboratory subjects are purposely doing whatever they can *to stay awake,* while the insomniac is doing whatever he can *to get to sleep.* However, these studies do offer us a useful, though perhaps exaggerated, picture of what most people experience as a result of common insomnia. That is, sleeplessness, or unsatisfactory sleep, puts a strain on the self-awareness circuitry. The circuits become "overburdened," so to speak.

The less efficiently you sleep, the less "with it" you tend to feel. Hence, nights of unsatisfying sleep are followed by days smattered with comments like, "I just can't think straight," "I can't keep my mind on what I'm doing," "I'm a little irritable today," "Would you mind repeating that? I just wasn't concentrating."

Cooling off + Cleaning up = Feeling "with it." That's what sleep is for.

How Sleep Works

The onset of sleep happens quickly. One minute you're awake and the next minute you're asleep. The complexity of biochemical and physiological events accompanying this shift from "awake" to "asleep" fills volumes of scientific works. However, for our purposes, we will view the mechanism of sleep in a general way.

Sleep is a natural, inborn inhibitory mechanism. It's a built-in protective response to prevent the "overheating" of your brain's energy circuitry. When the circuits are taxed to a certain point, a process of inhibition occurs. Although numerous electrophysiological changes are involved in this inhibitory process, I think we can assume that the big action takes place in the awareness energy circuitry. The reason we can make this assumption is because, from a practical point of view, the major difference between being awake and being asleep is the intensity of one's awareness.

So how does sleep happen? Something like this: 1) Your awareness energy circuits reach a point of "hotness"; 2) Simultaneously, your brain sends out "messages" to various organs and systems through your body; 3) The organs and systems make adjustments in response to these "sleep is needed" messages; 4) A process of inhibition occurs in your awareness energy circuits—they get ready to cool off; 5) Your self-anchoring imprint shifts from the "ON" to the "OFF" position so that the cooling off and cleaning up of sleep can get underway.

Although I have referred to your self-anchoring imprint as being in the "OFF" position during sleep, I am using the word loosely. As was stated previously in this chapter, your awareness doesn't totally shut down when you're sleeping; it's just relatively "off," relatively inactive, relatively disconnected. Furthermore, during the basic rhythmic cycle of sleep, variations in awareness levels occur. In the deepest states of sleep, your awareness is turned down to its lowest level. However, during other stages of sleep, your awareness moves closer to the surface, which accounts for your occasional ability to recall vivid dreams. These stages and levels of awareness are all part of the natural cooling-off/cleaning-up process of sleep.

The ability to sleep is something you're born with. It is not a special gift handed out to the lucky. Everyone sleeps. Therefore, everyone *can* sleep. Even if you're not sleeping well, you can feel somewhat confident knowing that you naturally possess all the necessary equipment and ingredients for bringing about a good night's sleep.

An Overview

Many of the concepts offered in this chapter will be applied to the solution of your sleep problem. Although there is no need to memorize any of this material, there are some general ideas you should keep in mind as you proceed through this book:

- Your brain is the "central control area" for all life's activities; real, electrochemical brain energy provides the power for everything you do.
- Your self-awareness energy circuits—those associated with your sense of self—are the highest nervous system energy use.
- Being awake is when the self-awareness energy circuits are in high gear; being asleep is when the self-awareness circuitry is relatively inhibited.

- The purpose of sleep is to cool off the self-awareness energy circuits and to clean up the imprint filing system (to integrate the newest information with the old). This rejuvenating process enables you to handle subsequent information efficiently—to feel "with it" each day.

- Sleep takes place when your self-anchoring imprint shifts from the "ON" position to the "OFF" position, relatively speaking.

❋   ❋   ❋

Sleep is an inborn mechanism everyone has. Insomnia is a problem a lot of people have. Unlike sleep, insomnia is not something you were born with. The next chapter will tell you how you got your sleeping problem, and what it really is.

5.

A PRACTICAL, UNMYSTERIOUS VIEW OF YOUR SLEEP PROBLEM

Let's go back to the time when you didn't have an insomnia problem.

Even then, you undoubtedly experienced a few restless nights here and there—nights when you were so excited about something, you couldn't wait for the next day to come, or nights when you were so upset about something, you just didn't think morning would ever come. Everyone has had those nights occasionally. And troublesome though they may be, such scattered episodes in your past were not enough to make you consider yourself an insomniac.

At some point along the way, however, a few restless nights started becoming a few too many restless nights as far as you were concerned. The scattered episodes were no longer the nights you couldn't sleep well; they were the nights you could sleep well. Thus, you began to consider yourself an insomniac, a person with an out-and-out sleep problem.

"Aha," many professional and lay advisers will say, "that's your whole problem in a nutshell. Your real problem is the fact that you view insomnia as a problem in the first place!"

Time and again I have heard and read of doctors advising insomniacs to "stop worrying" about their loss of sleep. "Accept your sleeplessness, and make the most of it," they tell bleary-eyed insomniacs. "Think of those extra waking hours as a gift rather than a curse."

Such advice is seldom greeted with enthusiasm. And for good reason—the advice is virtually useless. If you have a problem and need help, how helpful can it possibly be to be told, "You don't really have a problem, you just *think* you do!"? Not only is that kind of advice infuriating, but, practically speaking, there's nothing much you can do with it. Here's what one of my patients had to say on the subject when she first came to see me:

"I haven't had a good night's sleep in two years. A few weeks ago I decided the time had come to get some real help, not just another prescription for some tranquilizers or something like that. I wanted to find out what was really wrong with me and what I could do about it. So I made an appointment to see my doctor. He knew I'd been having some trouble sleeping because I'd casually mentioned it in the past. But this time I wasn't casual at all. I told him everything. Do you know what he said to me? He said,

'Don't lose any sleep over it.' I can't even tell you what I felt like saying at that point!"

Most doctors do not respond quite so callously to complaints of insomnia. However, even well-intentioned advice to "view insomnia as a blessing" is largely irrelevant. Anyone who says you don't really have a problem, when *you* say you *really do* have a problem, just doesn't know what a problem is.

A problem is not merely an "outlook" or a "frame of mind." It is much more tangible than that. Like everything else you experience, a problem is an imprint on your brain—an imprint linked by association to many other imprints.

Therefore, the problem of insomnia is a real, physical, tangible group of connected recordings in the storage area of your brain. Collectively, I will call all of these recordings a *can't sleep imprint.*

If you're having trouble sleeping, a *can't sleep imprint* is what you've got. Not a "psychological" problem. Not an "imaginary" problem. It is a *real* problem that exists as an imprint on your brain. The quality, action, and intensity of your imprint may not be the same as anyone else's, but the imprint is there, nonetheless.

If you want to start sleeping satisfactorily and awakening refreshed, it stands to reason that you've got to do something about that *can't sleep imprint.* Since you can't remove it surgically (even if you could, the potential risks would undeniably outweigh the benefits), the best alternative is to tone down the imprint—to refile it somewhere in the "back" near the "color-of-John-Doe's-tie" type of data.

In order to take the heat off your *can't sleep imprint,* you must first get to know this imprint of yours—how you ac-

quired it, how it grew, and how it operates. With this understanding, you will be ready to begin changing the imprint
(chapters 6, 7, 8). This chapter will help you pinpoint
what you'll be changing so that you can direct yourself to
Easy Sleep. If you're going to be successful at self-directing
a change, it's essential that you know what it is you're
changing.

The Night Before Christmas

Think back to that time in your life when you could
sleep relatively satisfactorily. Now search your memory
bank from those pre-insomnia days and see if you can recall
one of those nights when you couldn't sleep (e.g., the night
before you got married, the night before you left for a vacation, the night before a holiday). Even though you were
not an insomniac at that stage of your life, you did have occasional bouts of tossing and turning. Even young children
have these bouts. The words, "Mommy, I can't sleep," may
not be as common as the words, "Mommy, can I have a
drink of water?" But they do come up from time to time.

Recalling one of those sleepless nights from your past—
lets' say it was the night before Christmas—you certainly
had no expectation at that time of becoming a poor sleeper.
You did not have a habit problem of insomnia. But still,
something interfered with your natural inhibitory mechanism of sleep. Excitatory thinking, "the enemy of sleep,"
was the intruder.

Excitatory thinking is that overcharged kind of mental
activity you can't seem to control. When your mind is preoccupied with something, when you can't stop thinking
about something—that's excitatory thinking in action. It's

excessive, agitative, stimulatory mental activity. And "mental" though it may be, it is also *physical. Excitatory thinking is a physical use of your brain's energy*—your behavioral, self-awareness energy.

What causes excitatory thinking? The answer is change —*large change.* The change can take the form of an anticipated event, such as the night before Christmas. Or it can take the form of a past event, such as the night after winning the state lottery. In other words, it's not the *timing* of the change that counts so much as it is the *significance* of the change.

How do you judge the significance of a change? Every signal that comes into the energy power pack area of your brain represents a certain degree of change to your system. Just how much change the signal represents depends upon the amount of adjusting your brain has to do to integrate the new signal. For example, if you were to stick yourself with a pin accidentally, the sensation would immediately receive a large amount of concentrated energy from your awareness circuitry. A fairly intense imprint would then be recorded. However, because of what you've learned in the past, and because of the association links to previous imprints regarding the seriousness of the "injury," the sensation would quickly dampen down. Hence, the change represented by the pin prick would be small and you would adjust to it easily. On the other hand, if you broke your leg, the change represented by the injury would be large; greater adjustments would be required; the associated connections would be more far-reaching. The sensation caused by the broken leg would not dampen down quite so quickly and easily.

When faced with a relatively large change, you spend a good deal of time and energy thinking about the change—how it feels, what it means, what you'll do. With all of this "mental" activity going on, your self-awareness circuitry is in high gear. But, in order to sleep, the opposite is necessary: your self-awareness circuits must become relatively inhibited. If the circuits remain hot, busy, preoccupied, or excited, the natural inhibitory mechanism of sleep runs into a barrier.

Therefore, if you couldn't sleep the night before Christmas or the night after the lottery or whenever, the reason was that the event and its associated connections were occupying your self-awareness energy circuits overtime. Your energetic, excitatory thinking simply jammed the sleep mechanism.

During those pre-insomnia days of yours, sleep "jam-ups" were temporary and infrequent.

It may well have bothered you when you couldn't sleep, but the episode was usually forgotten by the next day or so. There was really no need to concern yourself with *why* you couldn't sleep the night before Christmas. Obviously, you were just too excited to sleep. Once the excitatory event had passed and the associated imprints had dampened down, you had no trouble sleeping.

The Excitatory Factor

Your present sleeping problem began with a "jam-up" similar to the night-before-Christmas situation. That is, it began with some significant change in your life—a change which threw you off balance, upset your equilibrium. What does it mean to be thrown off balance?

Every second of your life, your brain's energy systems are perpetually meeting the challenges of change. Every breath you take is a change; every word you hear is a change; every movement you make is a change. The multitude of changes, or stimulations, that come into your brain's power pack every day are actually the "food" that keeps your energy systems running. Thus, your brain thrives on changes, and it thrives on adjusting to changes. Brain activity is the electrochemical adjustments the brain constantly makes in response to changes. In terms of brain energy, there are essentially two ways in which your brain's systems can respond to change: they can respond in an excitatory ("doing") way, or they can respond in an inhibitory ("not doing") way. But, like a superb balancing act, these energy systems are always seeking to maintain an overall equilibrium between excitatory energy uses and inhibitory energy uses—between "activity" and "rest"—between "doing" and "not doing."

A significant change, however, will upset your brain's "balancing act." It will pose a greater challenge to your energy systems and will call for greater-than-average adjustments. The minute you become *aware* of the change—the minute you start *thinking* about it—your brain energy "scale" tips excessively toward the excitatory side in the behavioral energy area.

Needless to say, you cannot possibly go through life on an even keel. You inevitably have your ups and downs. But in most cases you adjust smoothly. Your brain has the capacity to adapt to almost any situation and re-establish a pattern of balance. Your night-before-Christmas excitement was certainly an instance of being out of balance; but without much effort at all, your brain soon re-established its normal balance.

Sometimes, however, certain changes can so throw you out of balance that you can't seem to make the necessary adjustments smoothly and easily. As you become progressively more preoccupied with the change, what you end up with is a lingering feeling of uneasiness which you can't quite shake off. Your growing awareness of your predicament further increases your excitatory energy imbalance, and insomnia is a common consequence.

Mrs. Brown: The Making of an Insomniac

To show, step-by-step, how a large change can result in insomnia, I'll now present a hypothetical case history. The story of "Mrs. Brown" is fictional, but any resemblance to the problems of real persons is purely intentional.

Mrs. Brown never had a sleeping problem until the day she received the news that her husband's business was relocating. The Browns would have to move to another state, and in anticipation of the move, Mrs. Brown experienced varying degrees of anxiety, excitement, and apprehension. The move would be a significant change for her. Giving up her house, her friends, her involvement in the community; finding a new home, packing and unpacking, making new friends and finding new activities—the thought of it all was unsettling, to say the least.

Looking beyond Mrs. Brown's feelings for a moment, what

went on in her brain at the time she was told "We're moving"? First of all, the news almost instantly received a large amount of energy from her brain's awareness circuitry; an intense imprint of "moving" was recorded in her brain.

Secondly, the news triggered off many old imprints by association. Memories of her last move 15 years before, unsureness about her ability to make new friends, thoughts about all the work ahead of her; numerous old imprints began playing back into her self-awareness circuitry.

And in addition, many old association connections in her brain were broken up and new associations began taking their place. The link between her name and her address, the link between her sense of purpose and her position in the community, the link between her present activities and her future plans—all of these associated imprints started changing. All in all, for Mrs. Brown, the anticipated change of moving caused an excessive amount of excitatory energy use. She immediately felt this imbalance as "agitation."

That first night after receiving the news, Mrs. Brown had a hard time falling asleep. She made various attempts to stop thinking about what lay ahead, but her efforts were in vain. Old imprints were playing back at such a high intensity that she could not overpower them by telling herself to calm down. Although her self-instruction to "calm down" also left an imprint on her brain, it wasn't strong enough to override the "moving" imprint and its associated thoughts and feelings.

By the time Mrs. Brown had experienced about five nights of wakefulness, the connection between her impending move and her new sleeping problem had grown stronger. Thus, a *can't sleep imprint* was now linked by association to an intense "moving" imprint.

As moving day grew near, Mrs. Brown became more and more concerned about her difficulty in falling asleep. Lying restlessly in bed, she would find herself thinking about all the work she still had to do, and how badly she needed her sleep. But, the more energy she focused on her sleeplessness, the stronger her *can't sleep imprint* became. To compound the problem, as her sleeping difficulty intensified, other signals became linked to her *can't sleep imprint*. These included the ticking of the clock, the darkness in the house, the feel of the sheets, the sight of her husband lying peacefully beside her. Numerous incoming signals occurring about the same time her *can't sleep imprint* was playing became associated with her sleeping problem. These signals had nothing to do with *causing* her sleep problem. They were "neutral" triggers. They merely became connected to her sleep problem because of a time link.

After the Browns had settled in their new community, the original cause of Mrs. Brown's sleeping problem—the anticipated move—was eliminated. Furthermore, she found it surprisingly easy to make friends and feel at home in her new environment. As far as she was concerned, there was no logical reason why she should still have trouble falling asleep. But she did have trouble. For, although the original stimulus for her insomnia was no longer a factor, her *can't sleep imprint* and many of its associated connections were still active recordings on her brain. To make matters worse, night after night, new imprint connections were added: the smell of fresh paint, the humming of the air conditioner, the color of the bedroom wallpaper, the swallowing of a pill, the clicking off of the television set, the setting of the alarm, etc., etc., etc.

What had evolved, unfortunately, was that by the time Mrs.

70

Brown had adjusted to the change of moving, she had already built up a significantly intense *can't sleep imprint*. Thus, when any one of the thousands of associated signals, such as the sight of her husband asleep, the setting of the alarm, etc., would come into her awareness circuitry, the signals would trigger off the unwanted wakeful response. Each night, as Mrs. Brown would settle into bed, she would automatically start feeling agitated, anxious, tense; she would find herself thinking excessively, despite her desire to control her excitatory thoughts and feelings. Satisfactory sleep eluded her.

Mrs. Brown, who never had a sleeping problem before she was faced with the change of moving, now had a habit problem of insomnia. The change of moving was past, but the excitatory brain energy activities associated with the change lingered on.

As time passed, Mrs. Brown no longer had any expectation of sleeping well. Experience had taught her that she couldn't. Her sincere efforts to conquer her insomnia—the milk, the drugs, the exercise—failed to help. Her efforts to understand *why* she couldn't sleep also failed to help. Was it some underlying neurosis? she wondered. Was it the "change of life"? Was she "unfulfilled"? The more she asked herself "why, why, why," the more confused, agitated and wakeful she became. Mrs. Brown was stuck and she had no idea of how it all happened.

The Vicious Circle of Insomnia

The making of an insomniac:

- It begins with a significant change in your life—a change causing excitatory feelings such as anxiety, agitation, uneasiness.

- The change leaves an intense imprint on your brain; old associated imprints ("memories") are retriggered; old association links give way to new ones.
- You become "preoccupied" with the change and its implications; you find yourself doing a lot of excitatory thinking. Thus, your self-anchoring imprint (your awareness) gets locked into the "ON" position, and the natural inhibitory mechanism of sleep is jammed.
- Although you may tell yourself to calm down or to think about something else, it doesn't seem to help. You're already using so much energy thinking about the change that your attempts to re-establish a balance aren't recorded with sufficient energy to override the intensity of your excitatory activities.
- Through repetition of this wakeful experience, a *can't sleep imprint* is formed in association with the big change you are going through. The more self-awareness energy you focus on the *can't sleep imprint*, the more intense it becomes.
- Even if you've made a reasonable adjustment to the change, your *can't sleep imprint* and numerous associated imprints can still remain intact.
- As you focus more and more of your concern on your sleeping problem, you constantly refuel the *can't sleep imprint*. You also pick up new association links along the way.
- Any of the association links, though they may be "neutral," can now trigger off the excitatory thinking, the uneasy feelings, the *can't sleep* response.
- Subsequent attempts and failures to solve your sleep

problem also become linked to your *can't sleep imprint.*
The whole predicament gets bigger instead of smaller.

*   *   *

The frustrating result: the more you think about the
problem and the harder you try to do something about it,
the worse it gets. To compound the dilemma, the more you
try *not* to think about the problem, the more you actually
are thinking about the problem, and the worse it gets . . .
like trying *not* to think about food when you're on a diet—
it's nearly impossible. Thus it doesn't seem to matter
whether you try to do something about your sleep problem
or you try *not* to do something about your sleep problem.
Either way, you end up focusing excessive energy *on* the
problem, thereby reinforcing the *can't sleep imprint.*

So there you have it, the vicious circle of insomnia.
*Everything you try to do to rid yourself of the problem ends
up becoming part of the problem.*

Those who advise you to stop worrying about your
insomnia, and to accept your sleeplessness and make the
most of it, are cognizant of the fact that excessive concern
about your problem isn't helping matters. But none of their
advice contains an adequate "how-to." *How* are you supposed to stop being overly concerned about it? . . . They
don't tell you, because they just don't know.

What few realize is that to solve your sleeping problem,
you actually have to change the intensity of your *can't
sleep imprint.* You have to break up some of the associated
connections that are automatically triggering it off. And
even fewer realize that *you*—and only *you*—have the capacity to do just that.

The Extent of Your Control

When you can't stop thinking about something—when you can't get something off your mind—how do you know you *can't?* You know because you've tried.

In the throes of insomnia, this "uncontrollable thinking" always occurs. There's always some neutral trigger around to set it off.

Naturally it's disturbing to lose control over any of your functions. But to lose control of your thought processes is disturbing in a different sort of way. *Thinking*, after all, is supposed to be a voluntary activity. You're supposed to be able to control it. Accepting that premise, you can't help but feel responsible and perhaps a bit guilty when you're unable to put an adequate rein on your thoughts.

The source of all this confusion and guilt is imbedded in the accepted definitions of "voluntary" and "involuntary." We generally assume, for example, that our internal organ activities are involuntary—beyond the scope of our deliberate control; nevertheless, we accept the fact that we can learn to control the functioning of our bowels and bladder at an early age. We also assume that our behavioral activities such as walking, talking, thinking, writing, etc., are voluntary—that we can and should be able to control them. Yet we readily accept the fact that we can lose control of a hand movement due to a muscle spasm.

We have inherited some rather artificial distinctions as to what constitutes a voluntary function and what constitutes an involuntary function. We also appear to have some vague criteria which allow for certain exceptions to the voluntary/involuntary "rule."

When it comes to thought processes, apparently such "exceptions" are rarely granted. It's difficult to prove, even in a court of law, that you're not *always* in control of your mental functioning. Yet during the course of an average day, everyone occasionally experiences indeliberate thoughts. Is there a person alive who is never distracted when some incoming signal triggers off an old memory? The sound of thunder, the aroma of coffee brewing, an old song on the radio—there's almost an infinite number of signals that cause people to get lost in their thoughts and to find their attention wandering.

In our traditional views about sleep, the artificiality of voluntary/involuntary distinctions is clearly demonstrated. We're taught, for example, that we can't make sleep happen. It's primarily an automatic, involuntary mechanism. But we're also taught that we must, to some extent, open the doors for sleep with a little voluntary preparation, like getting undressed, getting in bed, and getting comfortable. In addition, we learn that although we can't make sleep happen, we can make it *not* happen. We can deliberately postpone sleep for varying lengths of time. The distinctions between the voluntariness and involuntariness of sleep are already somewhat blurry. To blur them even further, we're taught that while we *can voluntarily* reduce our sleep, we *cannot involuntarily* reduce our sleep. In other words, if you purposely stay up all night, that's to your credit—but if you just can't fall asleep, it must be your fault.

There is only one meaningful way to determine what is

voluntary and what is involuntary, and that's on an individual basis. If you're in control of an activity, it's voluntary
for you. If you're not in control of an activity, it's happening
involuntarily. Whether you're talking about thought processes, feelings, or any other functions, if they're out of
your control, they're out of your control.

Hence, you are no more responsible for losing some control over your thought processes and ending up with insomnia than you are for losing control of your diaphragm
muscle and ending up with a bout of the hiccups. However,
given the proper tools, you can learn how to regain control
of your nighttime thoughts. You can learn how to take the
controls and direct yourself to sleep. And that truly will be
to your credit.

The Big Four Insomnia Categories

Trouble falling asleep, getting up frequently during the
night, getting up too early, not sleeping soundly—these are
the four most common insomnia problems. You can probably identify immediately with one of these categories. You
might even identify with more than one. But whether you
have one of the above or all of the above, the original source
of your insomnia was a significant change or series of
changes in your life. Although subsequent association links
have served to perpetuate your sleeping problem, *change*
was at its roots.

What is a significant life change? That depends entirely
on your point of view. What one person may view as a big
change, another may view as a minor change. A situation
you may adjust to quite easily, another individual may find

wrought with difficulty. The ease with which you adjust to any change depends on your past experiences, your present situation, your expectations, and countless other factors which make you different from everybody else.

Based on the case histories of numerous patients, here are some of the changes associated with the onset of sleeping difficulties. The precipitating events behind your insomnia might not be found in this list, but a glance at it may refresh your memory a bit. Brief patient descriptions follow:

- "My son turned 16 and got his driver's license."
- "My husband died."
- "My wife passed away."
- "I fell and broke my hip."
- "Final exams in college was the turning point."
- "I had surgery."
- "We had a baby."
- "I fell in love."
- "The doctors told me I had diabetes."
- "I was in an automobile accident."
- "For business reasons, I had to start traveling a lot."
- "I turned 50."
- "We moved to a new house."
- "I turned 65."
- "Our daughter got married."
- "I retired."
- "I found out my wife was cheating on me."
- "I found out my husband was cheating on me."
- "My back pain began."
- "The pressures at work got worse."

- "I was laid up in the hospital for two weeks."
- "I started my own business."
- "I quit smoking."
- "I was elected president of the school board."
- "I became very successful very fast."

Right now, you might not be able to point to a particular event in your past and say, "That's when my insomnia began." Your insomnia may not even relate to one big change in your life. It might have been a series of changes that cumulatively threw you off balance to the excessive excitatory side.

In any case, it's not vitally important to be able to identify the *exact* causal factor which precipitated your insomnia. Whatever the original trigger may have been, many other triggers have since become associated with your sleeplessness. It's quite possible that you long ago adjusted to that original causal factor. But whether you have or haven't, that *can't sleep imprint* can still remain as an active recording on your brain; any number of "neutral" triggers may be at work restimulating your habit of insomnia.

The important thing is not so much to identify the specific changes that may have started the ball rolling, but rather to understand how change in general can lead to insomnia. In other words, I'm not suggesting that there's some kind of "unresolved conflict" lurking in the depths of your subconscious mind and manifesting itself as sleeplessness. Even if there were some unresolved conflict that you could identify, there's no assurance that resolving the conflict would rid you of your sleeping problem. Getting at the roots of your problem and shouting "Eureka!" does not tell you how to solve your problem. It just tells you something about how you got your problem.

There are so many different kinds of changes that could result in insomnia that there's no absolute "cause-and-effect" rule applicable to everyone. Hence, to try to correlate certain kinds of changes with certain kinds of insomnia problems would be an exercise in futility. There is no definite correlation between the nature of a change and the nature of one's sleeplessness. You can't say, for example, that job changes always lead to difficulty in falling asleep, while 65th birthdays always lead to early morning awakenings. There are, however, some points worth mentioning about the development of the big four insomnia problems.

Falling Asleep

Jan, the 36-year-old teacher; Dorothy, the 62-year-old widow, and Bob, the 46-year-old executive were patients who had difficulty falling asleep.*

Jan, if you'll recall, traced her insomnia of four years duration back to the time she started teaching children with learning disabilities. The new job changed her life significantly. She immediately took her responsibilities seriously and felt a deep commitment to help the children. As a result, she found herself planning excessively, anticipating excessively, thinking excessively. And all this excitatory energy use kept her awake at night. Through repetition of the wakeful experience, her *can't sleep imprint* and its associated connections grew stronger. A falling asleep problem

---

* Patients discussed in these pages were previously mentioned in Chapter 1.

that started with a job change turned into a falling asleep problem that was triggered automatically, even on the weekends.

In Dorothy's case, it was the death of her husband that led to her insomnia. So many old association links were broken up. So many corresponding changes in her life resulted from her loss. Her initial difficulty in falling asleep was constantly retriggered every time she faced bedtime alone. Her excitatory feelings, characterized as *agitated depression*, were also restimulated nightly. Despite the admirable adjustment she had made in her daily life—she was busy, active, social—her sleep problem continually grew in intensity. Sleeping pills offered her only moderate relief. Dorothy's fear of thinking too much and of losing the kind of control she had managed to maintain during the day, served to reinforce her *can't sleep imprint*. The result was that her self-anchoring imprint, or self-awareness, was locked in the "ON" position. Initially, this "locking" may have been a deliberate means of avoiding depression. But after two years, there was nothing deliberate about her sleeplessness.

For Bob, the corporate product manager, it wasn't one change in particular that led to his difficulty falling asleep. It was the pressures of work in general—a loss of confidence in general, and perhaps a few "bad" decisions he had made. A vicious circle of insomnia had begun. Worrying about his position at work caused an excessive outpouring of excitatory energy use at bedtime; the worrying kept him awake ("ON"); the more concerned he became about his lack of sleep, the more wakeful he became; the more wakeful he became, the more he worried about his job. His *can't sleep imprint* and the constant changes and pressures of his executive position were intimately tied together, each one rekindling the other, day and night.

Looking at these three case histories, it is easy to see how a large change or series of changes can result in an increased use of the self-awareness circuitry and a corresponding increase in excitatory thinking. As the self-anchoring imprint gets locked on the change, the inhibitory mechanism of sleep is jammed. Then, through repetition of the sleeping difficulty, the *can't sleep imprint* is reinforced, and associated connections start serving as "neutral" triggers.

Falling asleep requires shifting off the day's activities and shifting off the worries and concerns that light up the self-awareness energy circuits. Excitatory thinking, which also includes *trying hard not to think,* prevents the easy occurrence of this shift from "awake" to "asleep."

Awakening During the Night

How does a pattern of awakening during the night evolve? Recalling Greg, 58, the hospital administrator, his insomnia began following his hospitalization for surgery. Although he had difficulty sleeping in the hospital due primarily to his anticipation of the surgery, his difficulty continued even after he recovered and returned home.

Hospitalization represents a significant change for most people. So much energy is concentrated on the situation that many imprints are strongly recorded throughout the ordeal. Anxieties, fears, sleeplessness, and sleeping pills all become linked by association. Even after the event is over, many of the imprints and associations can continue to exert their excitatory influence.

Greg's exploratory kidney surgery concluded with the removal of a benign cyst. He was well, he was healthy, he was greatly relieved. Nevertheless, he had been through a large change. Even the good news was a significant change. When he was released from the hospital and was home once again, that, too, was a change for him—another excitatory phenomenon which interfered with his sleep. Because of the association link between sleeping and pills, established in the hospital, Greg continued to take the sleeping medication. For numerous reasons (his expectations about tolerance, addiction, and other factors discussed in Chapter 3), the pills were no longer effective for him. Not only did he have trouble falling asleep, he also complained of awakening during the night. He related these arousals to nightmares, often pertaining to his hospitalization experience.

What had happened to Greg was that the large change of hospitalization had "jammed" the inhibitory mechanism of *staying asleep*.

During sleep's clean-up process (Chapter 4), the newest imprints—the ones that have received a proportionately large amount of awareness energy during the day—run back through the brain's energy circuitry. Older imprints linked by association also run through. Throughout the night, as the cleanup is going on, you normally go through stages ranging from *almost unaware* to *almost aware.**
Sometimes, however, if the imprints running through the

---

* In sleep research terms, the *almost unaware* stage would correlate to "Stage 4" or "delta" sleep (deep sleep); the *almost aware* stage would correlate to REM (rapid eye movement) sleep.

energy pool are sufficiently "hot" or if some external stimulus is sufficiently intense, it's possible to go one step further: you can go from *almost aware* to *aware*.

For Greg, it was the intense imprints associated with his surgery that would push him over the line from asleep to awake. After repeated episodes of awakening during the night, he had developed a habit pattern of interrupted sleep.

Getting up in the middle of the night doesn't have to go hand-in-hand with nightmares. Some patients attribute their awakenings to chronic pain problems. Others say they usually get up to go to the bathroom. And many say they're not quite sure what wakes them up.

But determining *what* has awakened you is really an after-the-fact exercise. For the *original* cause of this "can't sleep" problem is always some kind of change factor in your daily life—a change imprint that arouses you during its "cleanup." Your *subsequent* concern about the change, OR your concern about the sleep problem itself, serves to reinforce the pattern of interrupted sleep.

To sleep through the night, your self-anchoring imprint must remain relatively inhibited. However, since this vital imprint is linked to millions of other imprints, it can be triggered to the "ON" position by association, even during sleep. Sleep is, after all, an *active* state of the living human brain.

Getting Up Too Early

The story of Stan, 70, the retired policeman, fits the "early awakening" category of insomnia. Stan's problem began with the significant change of retirement, a change which affected his entire activity schedule, as well as his sense of purpose and direction.

The multitude of anxieties, apprehensions, and adjustments Stan experienced daily ran through his brain energy circuitry nightly. The result was a sleeping problem similar to that of awakening during the night. The large change Stan was going through jammed the inhibitory mechanism of *staying asleep*. Once his pattern of awakening at 4 A.M. was established, Stan couldn't seem to alter it, even when he went to bed later.

The significant difference between the person who gets up in the middle of the night and the person who gets up too early is that the former goes back to sleep, while the latter does not—he's up for the day. And what awakens the too-early riser? It could be anything from sunlight entering the bedroom to a realistic dream. As many sleep research studies have shown, deep sleep tends to occur in the first half of your night's sleep; in the second half, your sleep grows progressively lighter and your awareness moves closer and closer to the "surface." Thus, if your self-anchoring imprint isn't sufficiently inhibited, it doesn't take much to push your awareness "over the top." Once your self-anchoring imprint is "ON," all that excitatory thinking associated with the change can get underway and prevent returning to sleep.

Although Stan said he stayed in bed "thinking about things" at 4 A.M. because "there's nothing else to do at that hour of the morning," actually it was his thinking that prevented him from getting back to sleep. The thinking had become an automatic associated response that served to perpetuate his sleeping problem.

It's often said that early morning awakenings are correlated with the aging process—that the older you get the less sleep you need. Obviously, it's true that babies sleep more than adults. However, while on the average, total sleep time per 24 hours decreases by about 50 percent from infancy to young adulthood, the average remains the same from young adulthood to old age.

Although the *changes* and *expectations* associated with growing older may result in altered sleep patterns, this does not preclude elderly persons from learning how to re-establish desirable sleeping habits. In a 1976 report on the longevity and lifestyles of about 2,500 individuals, more than 1,000 persons ages 75 to 108 revealed that they slept between 7-½ and 7-¾ hours per night without difficulty.[1] Thus, aging and sleep loss don't have to go together. If a thousand elderly persons are sleeping efficiently, surely the potential exists for everyone.

Not Sleeping Soundly

The restless sleeper, the light sleeper, the unsound sleeper is the fourth big insomnia category. And it's Linda's category.

Linda was the 30-year-old artist and homemaker who hadn't slept well since the birth of her son, Billy. The baby represented an enormous change for Linda. And built right into that change was the fact that her sleep *had to be disrupted* for a while: the baby had to be fed, and Linda was the feeder. Like many parents, Linda became accustomed to awakening at the slightest noise from her baby. It wasn't long before her unsound sleep pattern was established. Sleeping "with one ear open," was how she described it.

With time, other association links were added to her problem, and her light sleep continued on for two years. Adding fuel to the fire were her worries and doubts as to how she could be a good artist, a good mother, and a poor sleeper at the same time.

The problem of light or unrefreshing sleep results when a significant change jams the inhibitory mechanism of sound sleep. In such cases, as you sleep, your self-anchoring imprint continues to play at a low frequency, but not low enough. Once again, the more concerned you become about your problem, the more intense your *can't sleep imprint* and its associated connections become.

* * *

Now that you have a new understanding as to how sleep problems can develop, it's time to start getting a handle on your own particular brand of insomnia. The following questionnaire will serve two purposes: 1) It will help you develop a clearer perspective about *your* sleep problem; 2) It will help you apply your understanding to the solution of your problem, as you will see in subsequent chapters.

Sleep Questionnaire

Questions 1–13 are designed to help you characterize your own sleep problem and its origins:

1) Do you have difficulty falling asleep?

2) Do you awaken during the night? If so, do you have any difficulty going back to sleep?

3) Are you troubled by early morning awakenings?

4) Are you troubled by unsound, fitful sleep?

5) Which of the following describe how you feel when you awaken?

  a) I feel listless, lethargic.

  b) I feel wide awake, refreshed.

  c) I'm groggy at first, but once I get going I feel all right.

  d) I'm irritable.

  e) Other.

6) During the day, do you feel fatigued?

7) Do you approach bedtime apprehensively? Calmly?

8) How long have you had a sleeping problem?

9) Has your sleep problem been chronic or intermittent?

10) If chronic, do you recall any significant changes in your life which occurred at approximately the same time as the onset of your sleep problem? (e.g.: injury, illness, marriage, divorce, a new baby, a new house, a job promotion or demotion, loss of a loved one, menopause, retirement)

11) If your sleeping problem occurs intermittently, can you recall the events surrounding its original occurrence? When your sleep problem started recurring, were there any changes in your life which coincided with the recurrence?

12) Have you sought relief from your insomnia through any of the following means?

  a) Sleeping medications

  b) Diet, exercise

  c) Therapy, psychological counseling

  d) Relaxation techniques, meditation

e) Dull books, warm baths, presleep rituals

f) Changes in bedtime schedules

g) Other

13) Did any of the above remedies bring relief? If so, what caused you to abandon the remedies or to look for other answers?

Questions 14–18 are designed to help you identify some of the associated activities and neutral triggers which may be perpetuating your insomnia:

14) During your daily life, do you find yourself thinking about:

a) The fact that you can't sleep?

b) The change or problem behind your insomnia (e.g. work pressures, family responsibilities, anticipated events)?

c) The ramifications of your sleeplessness, such as a lack of energy?

15) Do you discuss your sleep problem with family and friends? How do they tend to react to your problem? Do they inquire about your sleep?

16) Are there certain nights of the week or certain situations which seem to make your insomnia worse?

17) Do you notice any differences in your sleep patterns when you're on a business trip? A vacation?

18) Are there any external factors, such as noises, which seem to annoy you disproportionately at bedtime?

Answers to questions 19–20 will serve as specific aids in your practice of the Easy Sleep technique:

19) List at least three situations from your pre-insomnia

days in which you recall sleeping soundly and easily (e.g. sleeping in the back seat of your parents' car when you were a child; sleeping in a comfortable bed at a resort).

20) Based on your own experiences, list at least three situations which you find exceptionally relaxing, calming, and soothing (e.g. a concert in the park, a whirlpool bath).

6.

THE EASY SLEEP APPROACH—OR WHY YOU'LL BE DOING WHAT YOU'LL BE DOING

From this moment on, your past failures to solve your sleep problem no longer count. Even if you've tried and failed with 10 different medications, three yoga courses, a year of psychoanalysis, 50 gallons of milk, and every dull book in the library, you can now consider your record "clean." Whatever transient successes or failures you may have experienced in the past have occurred *in spite of you, not because of you.*

This time things will be different because YOU will be the one running the show. You will no longer be in the position of waiting for something to overpower you into "oblivion." Those kinds of approaches seldom work satisfactorily.

They are simply not as "powerful" as YOU are. But with you in the director's chair, with you in the position of controlling the events, you will be able to start accomplishing what you want to accomplish—efficient, rejuvenating, self-directed sleep. You *could not* have accomplished this before—not without an adequate "how-to." Now you can learn what that adequate "how-to" is all about. You can learn how such control can logically be your own.

What You "Can" Do

"There's no such word as *can't*," says the teacher to the pupil.

But, the teacher is mistaken. For, unless you are some sort of superman or superwoman, you have often concluded: *"I want to but I can't."* And when you've said it, you've meant it.

Of course, the rationale you would apply to that conclusion would vary significantly. If what you "can't do" is something you've learned *you're supposed to be able to do* (if it's considered voluntary), your reasoning might sound something like this: "I don't have enough will power," "I don't have the proper education," "I have too many other things on my mind." But, on the other hand, if what you can't do is something you've learned *you're not supposed to be able to do* (if it's considered involuntary), your rationale would sound more like this: "It's hereditary," "Medical science just hasn't done enough research yet," "It's physical."

There is certainly no reasonable person who would dispute the fact that certain events occur despite your wishes or efforts to the contrary. Undeniably, there are things over which you have little or no control, and it's really irrelevant whether you're "supposed to" have such control or not. What *is* relevant is that many activities which fall into the "I-want-to-but-I-can't" category are actually within the realm of your *potential control,* once you understand that YOU are part of an energy system. Not only are you part of it, YOU are the most vital, influential part of it. And YOU *can* control sleep. It is well within your potential.

To gain this control, however, you must overcome a barrier that has persisted through the ages. That barrier is the traditional confusion surrounding the meaning of the. word "you." It is a confusion that extends to many other words as well, such as "mind," "mental," "psychologic," "imaginary." All of these words historically have been linked to something that is somehow separated from everything else. Thus, we are constantly confronted with dualistic notions of "mental vs. physical," "real vs. imaginary," "you vs. your body," "mind vs. matter" and "mind over matter."

From what you have learned in the preceding chapters, I hope you now understand that mental *is* physical, that mind *is* matter, that *every* signal your brain receives is *real* no matter where the signal originates. When I speak of YOU or your thoughts or your imagination, therefore, I am talking about something very real. I am talking about the most important imprint on your brain—your self-anchoring imprint—and I am talking about the most complex uses of your brain's energy circuitry—your self-awareness, or thinking, activities.

You have already seen how your brain records all signals, linking and filing imprints in association with one another (see Chapter 4). As a result of this "association connection," what goes on in one "energy area" of your brain can effect a change in another "energy area of your brain. Your emotions can affect your autonomic activities; your autonomic activities can affect your behavior; your behavior can affect your emotions. All combinations are possible.

There is, however, only one way to *deliberately* effect a change in any area and that's through use of your self-awareness energy circuitry. Only YOU, with your sense of self, with your ability to self-direct events, can make things happen the way *you* want them to.

In Chapter 5 you saw how your awareness and concern regarding your sleep problem only serve to make matters worse. Now you will see how that same energy circuitry— your self-awareness circuitry—can be used to solve your sleep problem.

The Objectives

Right now you have a *can't sleep imprint* recorded in the *storage area* of your brain. You have a habit problem of insomnia. Through repetition of your problem, you also have numerous imprints that are linked by association to your *can't sleep imprint*. When restimulated, any of these associated imprints can play back into your brain's energy pool, thus triggering off your insomnia problem. Whether you have sleeping problems every night or only on Sundays or only when you stay in hotels or only on weekdays is not the determinant of whether or not you have a *can't sleep imprint*. If you feel you have a sleeping problem, that's proof enough that the imprint exists.

The first objective of the Easy Sleep approach, therefore, is to nullify the *can't sleep imprint* and to replace it with a *can sleep imprint*. Now, you may ask yourself, "How in the world can I put a *can sleep imprint* on my brain?" Remember, every single signal or stimulation you *ever* experience leaves an imprint on your brain. If you just say to yourself, "I can sleep," you are putting a *can sleep* recording on your brain (a weak imprint though it may be). Your words, thoughts, and ideas are *physical* stimulations—as physical as scratching your head. Every signal is real as far as your brain is concerned, no matter where the signal comes from.

The question, therefore, is not how to put an imprint on your brain—it's how to put an *intense enough* imprint on your brain. Telling yourself "I can sleep" leaves an imprint, but it's not strong enough to override the *can't sleep imprint*, which has been recorded with great intensity and has continued to build up through time.

To leave an intense *can sleep imprint* on your brain you must use an *energy concentration technique*. The reason: the more brain energy focused on an incoming signal, the more intensely the signal will be recorded. The Easy Sleep concentration technique, practiced in bed at night, enables you to harness a large amount of brain energy. It is your tool for directing "undiluted," concentrated energy on *can sleep* signals you will give yourself. Through the Easy Sleep technique, you will be able to form new, intense habit imprints of easy, efficient sleep. You will be able to turn sleep on and off at your direction.

The Easy Sleep approach has another objective as well. You might say it's a secondary objective, but it should not be overlooked. The objective is *getting more energy working for you during the day*. Although you most likely picked up this book in hopes of finding a solution to your insomnia, you of necessity had to have an additional motive in mind. Sure, it's lonely and frustrating to toss and turn all night. Given the choice, you'd prefer sleeping peacefully and soundly. But there's something more you're after: you would also like to have more energy to get things done when you're awake. So it's not just good sleep you're looking for—it's also some added energy-benefit of good sleep, a benefit now missing from your life.

To insure that you will get this added benefit of good sleep, your regular practice of the Easy Sleep concentration technique will be complemented with some corresponding daytime planning. As sleeping more efficiently will make you feel better when you're awake, using your waking hours more efficiently will help you sleep better at night.

Thus, the two objectives of Easy Sleep are *to direct yourself to a new habit of good sleep,* and *to derive the most benefit possible from the sleep you obtain.* Those are the goals. I will now explain how the Easy Sleep method is designed so you can reach those goals. Specific instructions will be given in Chapters 7 and 8. But before you get there, I want you to have a clear understanding of why you'll be doing what you'll be doing. In other words, you'll have more than a list of what-to-do's. You'll have the added and essential benefit of knowing how it all works. It must all seem *reasonable* to you, and not the least bit mysterious. After all, this is no "mind-over-matter" approach. This is a "your-mind-is-your-matter" approach.

The Principles of the Practice Technique

All of life's activities, whether excitatory or inhibitory in nature, are functional uses of energy—BRAIN ENERGY. The Easy Sleep concentration technique is your tool for gaining control of that energy so you can direct it toward obtaining satisfactory sleep.

There are three principal activities involved in practicing the technique: Relaxation, Concentration, and Imagination.

That doesn't sound very new, you might be thinking. You've been the "my-toes-are-sleeping-my-ankles-are-sleeping" route, but to no avail. You've tried concentrating on your breathing, and all you achieved were mild symptoms of hyperventilation. You've imagined yourself floating on clouds, but it hardly captivated your thoughts. None of those "tricks" ever worked before, so why should any of them work now?

First of all, there are no tricks involved in the Easy Sleep technique. The Easy Sleep technique works because it's a tool for *self-directing sleep*. When you're directing events, your results cannot possibly be tricky. Secondly, there are *fundamental differences* between the Easy Sleep technique and other so-called relaxation/meditation exercises. Among the most important differences are:

1) The Easy Sleep technique uses relaxation, concentration, and imagination as vehicles for self-directing a change in your

brain; other techniques employ these activities for their soporific or calming effects only.

2) The Easy Sleep technique emphasizes your *active* participation in its practice; other techniques require that you maintain a passive attitude at all times.

3) The Easy Sleep method requires both practicing the technique and understanding the principles behind what you're practicing; other techniques emphasize practice, but overlook the importance of your understanding.

Essentially, when you practice the Easy Sleep technique you will be an active, informed participant directing your brain's energy to obtain and maintain satisfying sleep. The three principal activities, Relaxation, Concentration, and Imagination, aren't designed simply to lull you to sleep. Each one of the activities plays a logical, tangible role in helping you change from a "can't sleep" person to a "can sleep" person, as I'll now explain.

The Role of Relaxation

Make a fist with your right hand. Clench it as tightly as you can. You can readily experience the tremendous amount of energy it takes to keep your fist clenched. As you tighten your fist, it becomes more difficult to concentrate on what you're reading. The reason, quite simply, is that you're splitting your brain energy between reading the book and maintaining your tightly clenched fist.

Now loosen your fist and let your hand go limp, relaxed. You feel relieved. You also find it easier to concentrate on the words in front of you.

The Easy Sleep technique involves muscle relaxation because relaxation facilitates concentration. As you release excess tension from your peripheral muscles during your practice of the technique, you will have more energy available to use at your direction.

Muscle relaxation also facilitates a better brain energy balance. As you saw in the preceding chapter, wakefulness results from excessive excitatory brain energy use. This "excitatory factor" manifests itself as anxiety, tension, uneasiness, agitated thinking, worrying, etc. By relaxing your muscles, you are helping to reduce excess tension. You are alleviating some of the excitatory activity that contributes to your wakefulness.

Taut muscles "split" brain energy, thereby making it more difficult to accomplish what you want to accomplish. Taut muscles also contribute to brain energy imbalances, thereby making it more difficult to tone down some of that excessive excitatory activity that keeps you awake.

Relaxation means more brain energy working for you, more energy available to use at your own direction. When the desired direction is satisfying sleep, muscle relaxation expedites arriving at the destination.

The Role of Concentration

In Chapter 5 you learned that your sleeping problem is an imprint on your brain. For simplicity, we called this a *can't sleep imprint*. You also saw how any number of signals or stimulations can trigger off your *can't sleep imprint* and its associated excitatory activities, such as excessive thinking, worrying, feelings of anxiety, etc.

That you *want* to change your present habit of insomnia is indisputable; that you *want* to quiet those excitatory activities that keep you up is also indisputable. But *wanting* to make this desirable change and *actually making it* are two different things. *Wanting* is simply not powerful enough to facilitate the change. The power comes from concentration. Why is this so?

Because of brain energy. All imprints are recorded on your brain with a certain amount of energy—a certain degree of intensity. For purposes of illustration, let's use a power term and say that through repeated episodes of insomnia, you have a *can't sleep imprint* of "10 watts."

Now suppose that while lying in bed, your wheels are spinning a mile a minute as you think and worry about one thing or another. Since you want to get to sleep, you might then give yourself some positive suggestion such as, "I will fall asleep soon" or "I will stop worrying about what I have to do tomorrow" or "I *can* sleep." Your suggestion would certainly leave an imprint on your brain. But, because you are feeling tense and you're aware of numerous distractions, your brain energy would be "split," as it was when you tried clenching your fist and reading at the same time. In other words, your brain energy would not be concentrated in any one area. Your positive suggestion, as a result, would receive only "1 watt" of energy, leaving a "1 watt" imprint—not strong enough to overpower the "10 watt" *can't sleep imprint.*

However, if your body were relaxed and you were relatively undistracted, you would have more energy available to concentrate on the suggestion or signal you'd give yourself. A suggestion given in a concentrated state leaves a far stronger imprint on your brain than a suggestion given in an unconcentrated state.

Hence, when your brain's energy is concentrated, you can boost up a "1 watt" suggestion. You can magnify it to 15 or 20 watts and derive a 15- or 20-watt effect. That's the power of concentration.

The power of concentration and the power of change are intimately tied together. Recalling that significant change, or series of changes, that led to your sleep problem, it becomes apparent that the larger a change, the more energy you focus on it. *Significant change concentrates energy*. Furthermore, in a concentrated state, other incoming signals occurring at approximately the same time as the change also receive a large amount of energy. Numerous intense imprints thus become linked to the change by association.

An example of how large change concentrates energy is the old pie-in-the-face routine: an unsuspecting "victim" is casually engaged in conversation when his "buddy" whips out the pie and . . . Wham! Big change! The victim suddenly feels the whipped cream dripping from his face, and the whole scene takes on a new meaning. His brain's self-awareness energy circuitry immediately circles in on the pie, the feel of it, the taste, the mess, and last but not least, the "pie-thrower," his so-called "buddy." This event leaves intense imprints on the victim's brain, and although he may learn to laugh about it later, he won't soon forget any of it.

Clearly, changes that *happen to you* have the capacity to concentrate your brain's energy and leave strong impressions, or imprints, on your brain. But suppose *you* want to make a significant change happen? Suppose *you* want to make the change from an insomniac to an Easy Sleeper? Since you can't wait for someone to do something like throw a pie in your face, you'll have to concentrate your brain's energy yourself.

Everyone, of course, complains at one time or another of an inability to concentrate. It's a common problem we all encounter in our daily life. The Easy Sleep method is designed specifically to overcome this particular obstacle. Obviously, if you knew how to concentrate on whatever you wanted to concentrate on, you wouldn't have much of a sleeping problem. You'd just "think about something else" when some excitatory thought was keeping you awake. But as I said earlier in this book, controlling your thoughts is a lot easier said than done. You must have some practical steps for accomplishing that kind of feat.

The Easy Sleep technique provides you with those practical steps, as you will see in forthcoming chapters. For now, the important thing is to understand why concentration is essential to making a desirable change. To review: when your brain's energy is concentrated rather than split, a suggestion or signal you give yourself will leave a strong, intense imprint on your brain.

The Role of Imagination

Imagined events have always been associated with the nonphysical, the intangible, the unreal. "It's just your imagination," it's often said. The implication is that if you're imagining something, you're either living in a dream world, you're a hypochondriac, you're out-of-touch, you're paranoid, you're pretending, or you're engaging in a little harm-less fantasy. Whatever the explanation may be, the act of imagining is almost always looked upon as an activity that isn't really real.

But, your imagination *is* real. An imagined experience, like any other experience, is a brain energy event, leaving a brain energy imprint. When you close your eyes and form a visual image of something, you're actually picking and choosing past-recorded imprints from your memory bank and playing them back through your self-awareness energy circuitry. Although derived from past-recorded signals, the imagined event is amplified and imprinted on your brain just as any new incoming signal would be.

Not only is an imagined event a real, electrochemical brain energy occurrence, but its effects can also be quite real. Imagining an experience can affect your behavior, your emotions and your autonomic functions in the same way that "living" an experience can.

Suppose, for example, that you are waiting to meet a friend for dinner and she is already well over an hour late. As the minutes pass by, you say to yourself, "I can't imagine what's keeping her. She's never late." But, you *can and do* start imagining all sorts of possibilities. And, eventually, you find yourself imagining the worst: your friend must have been in some terrible accident. The imagined accident makes you feel panicky—a *real*, emotional response. It causes you to light up a cigarette or pace the floor—a *real* behavioral response. And it causes an increase in your pulse and breathing rate—a *real* autonomic response. When your friend finally shows up, you don't know whether to kiss her or "kill" her. You have been through a harrowing experience. But it was *"just your imagination."*

As you saw in Chapter 4, *every* signal, or stimulation, you receive leaves an imprint on your brain with the capacity to play back into your energy power pack area. But the intensity of an imprint and its playback are not governed by how externally real vs. imaginary the signal may be. The intensity and significance of a signal are a function of 1) the amount of brain energy focused on the signal, and 2) the associated imprints triggered by the signal.

Thus, imagining your friend in an accident could cause you to react *as if* you had actually received word of an accident. Although you would not necessarily react the *same way* in both instances, your reactions would be real in either case.

To imagine something is to think something. And thinking, of course, is what's keeping you up—excitatory, uncontrolled thinking. When you practice the Easy Sleep technique, you will also be thinking, but your thoughts will be *controlled, concentrated,* and *calming.* Through the creative, concentrated use of your imagination, you will be able to form strong, new imprints that say *can sleep.*

❂   ❂   ❂

Relaxation, Concentration, and Imagination are the three principal activities involved in the Easy Sleep technique. Although I have discussed each activity separately, they do in fact work simultaneously, complementing each other.

As you are relaxing your muscles, for example, you will also be concentrating on your muscles and imagining that you see them relaxing and unwinding. Similarly, as you concentrate your energy on an image, you will also be enhancing your relaxation. And, as you imagine words or scenes, you will be enhancing your concentration, giving it a focal point.

The Easy Sleep concentration technique is designed to help you achieve a new, intense imprint of *can sleep.* Through Relaxation, Concentration, and Imagination, you can gain control of your thought system. You can shift your self-awareness off of the complex of activities that are jamming the natural inhibitory mechanism of sleep.

Once again, in brief, this is how the three principal activities work together:

- By relaxing your muscles, you are gathering up brain energy—extra energy that you'll need for self-directing a change in your sleep habit.
- By concentrating this brain energy, you can increase the power or intensity of any "message" you give yourself.
- By using your imagination, you can focus your concentrated energy on specific *can sleep* thoughts and experiences which are then strongly imprinted on your brain.

The Easy Sleep concentration technique will give you experience at self-directing your thoughts, and hence, your sleep. As you steadily gain this experience, you'll also steadily advance your new expectation that you *can* assume control where you couldn't before. Day by day, the reasonableness of self-directed, refreshing sleep will become more and more apparent to you.

To enhance the daily benefits of refreshing sleep even

further, a little daytime planning for "energy conservation" is called for.

The Principles of Daytime Planning

Your sleeping problem is now consuming a portion of your daily energy. In some ways, it is consuming a disproportionate amount of your daily energy. This is not your fault; it is part of the whole vicious circle of insomnia.

When you don't sleep well at night, it robs you of energy you'd like to have during the day. Added to this, your understandable daily concern over your sleep problem further depletes your already depleted supply of energy. To make matters still worse, the more you focus on your problem and its implications during the day, the more you inadvertently reinforce your insomnia at night.

To solve this circular "energy crisis" you must practice the Easy Sleep technique nightly. But you'll also have to rechannel some of that energy you're now using as you think and worry about your problem during the day. For, as you well know, focusing excessive awareness on your problem only serves to make matters worse.

The way to rechannel that daily energy is by planning and instituting some new activity. Bah! you say—it's hard enough to handle your present activities. Bah! you say— you don't need to change your *life*—you just want to sleep better. Bah! you say—you have neither the time nor inclination to start something new—you rarely finish what you start, anyway.

In answer: First of all, I know it's hard enough handling your present activity schedule. The principles of daytime planning are there to make it easier. Secondly, I am not suggesting you need to "change your life." The principles of daytime planning are intended to help you *sleep better.* Thirdly, you *will* have the time and inclination to start something new once you begin practicing the Easy Sleep technique. You'll also have the energy to continue with and finish what you start. The principles of daytime planning are there *to make you feel better and sleep better.*

As to what you will plan and what you will do, Chapter 8 will help you decide. But whatever you choose, the new activity will definitely be something *you want* to do. It will not be a chore or a burden. Look at it this way: Right now you are using up energy during the day by thinking about your sleep, or your lack of it. Certainly, you don't *want* to use your energy this way, nor do you *enjoy* using it this way. Wouldn't you rather use that energy doing something you want to do—something you enjoy doing? And wouldn't it be gratifying if you found that doing this new "thing" also enhanced your sleep?

The new daytime activity will be *your* time. You'll select the activity. You'll institute it. And most importantly, you'll derive immediate daily and nightly benefits from it. It will make Easy Sleep a lot easier.

New Odds and New Plans

With your new perspective of your sleep problem and your new understanding of how the Easy Sleep method works, you can now approach your solution with a reasonable expectation of success. Remember, expectations, like thoughts, words, and images, are physical imprints recorded in the storage area of your brain.

Your new expectation, which will continue to grow stronger, should sound something like this:

"I have a tremendous amount of brain energy to use at my direction. As I practice the Easy Sleep concentration technique, I can now reasonably expect to change my habit imprint of *can't sleep* and to replace it with a strong imprint of *can sleep*. I can reasonably expect to direct myself to fall asleep, sleep efficiently, and awaken in the morning feeling alert and refreshed."

In conjunction with your new expectation about sleeping better, you can also begin to expect that you'll feel more energetic during the day. For, not only will you be forming a new *can sleep imprint*, but you'll also be using your daily energy more efficiently. By planning new activities during your waking time, you will have a shorter distance to go when it is sleeping time. Plus, you'll get more mileage from your sleep.

Satisfying sleep—what was once a long shot for you—is now a good bet. The odds are overwhelmingly on your side.

7.

PRACTICE STEPS
FOR
EASY SLEEP

You can now bid the unreliable sandman and all those elusive sleep panaceas an official goodbye. As you'll soon discover, the most effective and dependable sleeping agent is *you*.

The Easy Sleep concentration technique you're about to learn will be your *central* instrument for obtaining satisfying sleep at your own direction. The technique is the master tool for climbing out of that position of helplessness and into a position of *control*. So . . . Goodbye, Sandman—Hello, YOU!

* * *

As you saw in the last chapter, the Easy Sleep technique involves Relaxation, Concentration, and Imagination.

These activities are the fundamental components of self-directed sleep. To review, the three principal activities enable you to:

1) Gain control of a significant amount of brain energy—energy that was "split" before;

2) Use that concentrated energy to form strong new imprints and associations that say *can sleep;*

3) Produce a more desirable brain energy balance by reducing some of your excitatory energy use;

4) Direct your self-awareness circuitry off of what's keeping you up and onto what "cools" you down.

The Easy Sleep technique is designed to obtain better sleep as soon as possible, AND it's also designed to obtain a new habit of satisfying sleep—a habit that will LAST.

In this chapter, I'll begin with general instructions for practicing the basic Easy Sleep concentration technique. Following these instructions, I will offer suggestions for adapting the technique to the "big four" insomnia problems: difficulty falling asleep, early morning awakenings, getting up during the night, and unsound sleep. Special questions regarding the technique will be handled at the end of the chapter.

Practice Setting

The Easy Sleep technique is practiced in bed. But, before getting in bed, take whatever steps you deem necessary for making your surroundings as peaceful as possible.

For example, you might want to adjust the temperature

in your room by opening a window or resetting the thermostat. Or, if you happen to be a habitual clock-watcher who anxiously keeps track of the number of hours remaining before wake-up time, you might make it easier on yourself by turning the clock around so you can't see its face. If various noises tend to disturb you, you may wish to turn on a fan or some other appliance that will provide a constant background sound.

Do whatever you can reasonably do to keep exterior distractions to a minimum. Naturally, there may be some distracting elements you can't do much about at this point, but through your practice such distractions will become minimal. For now, just arrange things as well as you can to provide for your own comfort.

Practice Length

The Easy Sleep technique must be practiced *every* night, preferably at bedtime. Initially, while you're getting used to the technique, plan on practicing for *about* 15 minutes nightly. Depending upon the nature and intensity of your sleep problem, you may find that you need a few minutes more or less than this 15-minute average. If your difficulty is falling asleep, for example, it may take you a little longer than the average for a few nights. If, on the other hand, your difficulty is staying asleep, you may find that you can manage to practice for only five or ten minutes before sleep. But you may need to repeat your practice if you should awaken at some undesirable hour. Later in this chapter, these time variations will be explained in greater detail.

As you become more proficient at using the technique, you'll be able to cut down your practice time considerably. Eventually, after your desired sleep pattern is well-established, you can graduate to the abbreviated Easy Sleep mini-technique for maintenance (Chapter 9). But before you can maintain your habit of efficient sleep, you've got to develop it, and that usually entails about 15 minutes of practice nightly.

How Many Nights It Takes

There is absolutely no way for me to judge the intensity of your particular sleep problem. Therefore, I cannot give you a meaningful prediction as to how many nights of practice it will take before you start getting the kind of results you're looking for. Some people get results the first time they use the technique. Others require a week or more before their sleeping pattern improves significantly. But whether it takes you a few nights or a few weeks to reach your goal, the important thing is: you will reach it. Everytime you practice the technique you are helping to break up old patterns of poor sleep. Every time you practice the technique you are helping to establish a better brain energy balance. And, every time you practice the technique you will be moving closer to a real, lasting solution to your sleep problem.

After you have succeeded in obtaining the kind of night's sleep you want, you'll need some time to reinforce your desirable sleep pattern. Therefore, for approximately *30 days following your initial success,* continue to practice the basic Easy Sleep concentration technique described in this chapter. This additional practice will be your best insurance of continued success, as it will help intensify your new *can sleep imprint*.

The Practice Steps

Positioning Yourself

With distractions to a minimum, get in bed and lie on your back. Prop your head up with a few pillows, and be sure that your arms and legs are uncrossed. When you feel you are in a comfortable position, close your eyes.

Note: If for any reason you cannot lie comfortably on your back, assume a position that is most comfortable for you. If possible, find a position that is different from the one in which you usually sleep.

Step One: Unwinding

Now that you are in your comfortable position, you will begin to relax your muscles, starting from the top of your head and working all the way down to the tips of your toes. As you tell yourself to relax each muscle group, imagine that you see the muscles unwinding, uncoiling, and releasing tension.

What follows is a sample Unwinding exercise. Read this exercise a few times until you feel you are familiar with the basic process. You don't have to memorize the words; just get the idea of what you'll be telling yourself to do when you Unwind.

Sample: "Relax. And let yourself go. Feeling all that tension uncoil from your muscle fibers. Relaxing your scalp muscles. Moving down to your face muscles. Now wiggle your tongue, loosen it, let it lie flat on the floor of your mouth. Now feeling that relaxation spread to all the muscles around the mouth, letting the corners come up. As you release the tightness in your eye-balls, you let them roll up under your lids . . . no longer posed for reading and thinking on the day's events. Now feeling that relaxation spreading down to your neck muscles and your shoulder muscles. All that tension unwinding and spreading a tingling sensation from the tops of your arms to your elbows, to the very tips of your fingers. The tingling sensation gives way to a feeling of lightness and your arms feel so loose and so re-laxed.

"Now feeling that relaxation spreading from your chest . . . to your back . . . to your abdomen . . . to your trunk muscles. And you feel so much better. So much calmer. Layer upon layer of tension removed. The tightness now unwinding from your thigh muscles . . . down to your knees . . . your calves . . . your feet . . . and to the tips of your toes. All the muscles of your legs feel so relaxed, so loose. You take a deep breath now—all the way in and all the way out—releasing that last little bit of surface ten-sion. And you feel so good. So peaceful. So calm."

The Unwinding phase of the Easy Sleep technique should take you about five minutes to complete. With a little experience, you'll be able to tell when your body feels relaxed. The sample exercise talks about a feeling of "light-ness" in the muscles, but you may find that your muscles feel "pleasantly heavy" when you're relaxed. Or, you may describe your relaxed feeling as a "general warmth." How-ever you choose to describe your feeling of relaxation, you will be the best judge of determining when you have completed the Unwinding phase. It may take you more or less than five minutes to Unwind, depending upon how tense you feel before you begin. The time factor not only varies from one individual to another, but it also may vary from one day to another in any given person.

There are two additional points that should be made about the Unwinding phase:

1) As long as you unwind your muscles in the general direction of *head to toe*, the order of relaxing specific muscle groups can be altered. For example, you can relax your chest and back muscles before your arm muscles, or you can relax your abdominal muscles before your back muscles, etc. All you need to remember is to start from the top and work your way down. With this pattern in mind, slight variations in the order of relaxation are perfectly acceptable.

2) When you start your Unwinding exercise, be sure to loosen your tongue and to roll your eyes slightly upward. These brief measures will immediately help you to break off some of those excitatory thoughts that interfere with your sleep.

By loosening your tongue, you are releasing it from that tight, ready-to-talk position associated with your daily activities and concerns.

Similarly, by rolling your eyes upward beneath your lids, as if you were looking at your forehead, you are releasing them from their intense, reading-and-seeing, daytime position. As you continue through the other phases of the Easy Sleep technique, your eyes may roll back down quite naturally. However, if you find yourself distracted at any time throughout your practice—if you find your thoughts wandering back to the problems and concerns of daily living—roll your eyes up again momentarily. It will enable you to break your unwanted train of thought easily.

The eye roll procedure is a vital tool that can be used again and again as you practice the Easy Sleep concentration technique. It is one sure way of quickly disconnecting that uncontrolled, excitatory thinking. So if you find your thoughts getting off the track, a little eye roll will help you get back on the right track—the track towards "easy sleep."

Once you have spread that relaxation from the top of your head all the way down to the tips of your toes, you are ready to go on to Step Two of the Easy Sleep technique.

Step Two: Directing

With all that excess energy released from your peripheral muscles, you will have succeeded in harnessing a good deal of your brain's energy. You can now direct this "unsplit" concentrated energy on forming new imprints and associations that say *can sleep.*

In your calm, relaxed state, what you'll now do is *imagine yourself getting the kind of night's sleep you want.* Remember, as far as your brain is concerned, an imagined event is just as *real,* just as *physical,* as any other event. So by Directing your concentrated brain energy on an imaginary scene, you are actually forming new imprints in the storage area of your brain. You are actually putting in a new group of recordings or messages more to your liking. As you form a new image of yourself sleeping "in your mind's eye," you are breaking up those old associated *can't sleep* connections and are replacing them with new imprints of *can sleep.*

Essentially, all you have to do is imagine yourself sleeping comfortably and satisfactorily and waking up at the time you desire, feeling alert and refreshed. Because you will be using your imagination in a concentrated state, your brain will record the scene with sufficient energy to form intense imprints. Hence, through use of your imagination, you can direct a significant, desirable change in your habit patterns.

Here are some sample Directing scenes you can imagine during Step Two. You can, of course, invent your own:

Imaginary Scene: You are sleeping soundly throughout the night. You awaken in the morning and have a new feeling of invigoration. As the sun drifts into your room, you look at your clock and smile with satisfaction. It's just the time you planned on getting up. You stretch with pleasure and get out of bed. You feel so good. You are ready to start a new day.

Imaginary Scene: You see sleep as a rejuvenating process which occurs for the sole purpose of serving YOU. It has only one important function—giving that great, complex mind of yours a chance to rest and freshen up. You feel very good knowing that your daily intellectual functioning is so awesome that it requires time off for rest and rejuvenation. You smile as you see sleep get underway, cooling off and cleaning up your self-awareness circuitry. You marvel at how efficiently and confidently the job of sleep proceeds. Throughout the night, your body's energy systems are maintaining a perfect balance while your mind is getting in gear for the next day. In the morning, you awaken feeling alert, refreshed and re-energized.

Imaginary Scene: Turning your time clock back a few years, you recall a wonderful vacation you once had. You felt so good on that vacation—so carefree and happy. After each enjoyable day, you'd feel pleasantly exhausted. Contentedly, you'd climb into that comfortable bed with the cool clean sheets. Flicking off the light, you'd lie back, feeling so relaxed, thinking only of more pleasant and carefree days to follow. In the mornings, you'd awaken with a true zest for living. As you recreate this scene, imagine sleeping just that comfortably and awakening just that refreshed tonight, tomorrow, and every night.

Imaginary Scene: You are sleeping with a slight smile on your face. It is a smile of self-assurance, for you know you're getting a good night's sleep—that your energy systems are being recharged for the next day. You see your arms and legs move occasionally . . . you change positions from time to time . . . and it is all so satisfying. You awaken in the morning and have a few minutes to relax in bed before getting up to dress. You stretch your muscles, and all traces of grogginess vanish. You get out of bed and feel positive about yourself.

The Directing phase of the Easy Sleep technique should take you only about two or three minutes to complete. But you needn't clock yourself. Take as much time as you please before moving on to Step Three.

Note: When you are directing your imaginary scene, remember to employ the eye roll device if you should find yourself distracted by unwanted thoughts or feelings. Let your eyes roll up for a few seconds, and then continue on with your practice.

Step Three: Drifting

Now that you have directed your concentrated energy on forming a new *can sleep imprint,* you are ready to begin the final phase of the Easy Sleep technique. The purpose of the Drifting phase is to promote the inhibitory process that will lead naturally into sleep.

During this phase, you will once again construct an imaginary scene. But view the transition between Steps Two and Three as a fading out of one scene and a fading in of the next. In other words, your Step Two Directing scene should lead gracefully into your Step Three Drifting scene.

The imaginary scene you'll construct in this phase of the technique should be a comfortable, relaxing, secure setting with you at the center of the scenery. Imagine yourself experiencing all the pleasant sensations that the scene would elicit. Your overall feeling should be one of drifting or moving peacefully through the scene.

Sample Scene: You are lying on a soft grassy knoll by the edge of a shallow, clear brook. It is a beautiful summer day and the sun is shining through the rich green of the trees above you. You feel so calm as a gentle breeze touches you. The constant sound of the brook water rippling over the glistening rocks is so relaxing that you begin to feel as if you were part of the gentle motion. The fresh air, the smell of the greenery, the sounds of the water, the feel of the velvety grass and the breeze are all so refreshing, they make you tingle with peaceful pleasure. You feel yourself drifting deeper and deeper into the relaxing, enveloping scenery.

Some other ideas for imaginary Drifting scenes are:

- Rocking in a cozy chair by a fireplace at a ski lodge.
- Sitting by the shore at the beach, as the waves roll softly back and forth.
- Taking a carriage ride on a spring day.
- Lying on a couch and watching TV, as someone gently scratches your back.
- Floating on a big raft in a swimming pool.
- Relaxing on a porch swing on a summer evening.

You can choose any kind of imaginary scene that appeals to you. It can be a scene based on a past experience or it can be totally "fictional." If you desire, you can use your imagination to shift from one scene to another. You may also wish to construct a more active scene than those I've suggested. For example, you can imagine yourself swinging a golf club effortlessly and rhythmically, or you can see yourself calmly hitting one tennis ball after another with the "sweet spot" of your racket.

The basic idea of your Drifting scene is to focus your imagination on something that is sensually satisfying, calming, and pleasantly monotonous. Once you become involved in the scene, you will probably fall asleep quite soon. As sleep comes on, you will naturally and effortlessly assume your sleeping position. You don't have to make a point of remembering to do this. It's already part of your built-in expectation. When sleep begins, you'll find yourself just getting into the most suitable position without even trying.

If you are practicing your Drifting scene but still find yourself wakeful, your imagination is probably wandering off the scene and onto those excitatory thoughts. So, the first thing to do is to roll your eyes up to break the unwanted thought activity. Next, either go back to the scene you were "in," or start another one. You can employ the eye roll as often as you need to, and you can change the scene as often as you like.

As you become more proficient at using the Easy Sleep technique, you'll find it easier and easier to drift off to sleep during Step Three. The way to become more proficient is through practice—regular, nightly practice. If you follow the steps and practice regularly, you'll see improvement in a matter of nights.

The Basic Technique and the Big Four Problems

There is one basic Easy Sleep concentration technique, and that's the one just described in this chapter. To review:

Preparation: With distractions to a minimum, get in bed; lie on your back; elevate your head with some pillows, and be sure your arms and legs are uncrossed.

Step One (Unwinding): Relax your muscles, group by group, from the top of your head to the tips of your toes. As you Unwind, imagine seeing the tension leaving your muscles. Be sure to loosen your tongue and roll your eyes upward at the beginning of this step. Once your muscles are relaxed, you will have more energy available to use at your direction.

Step Two (Directing): To form new, intense *can sleep* imprints Direct your concentrated energy on seeing yourself getting the kind of night's sleep you want. Picture yourself sleeping efficiently and awakening at the time you desire, feeling alert and refreshed.

Step Three (Drifting): To promote the process of inhibition, and to turn sleep on, construct a comfortable, sensually satisfying, pleasantly monotonous scene in your mind's eye. Imagine yourself Drifting peacefully through the calming, soothing scene.

❊ ❊ ❊

These three steps—Unwinding, Directing, and Drifting —form the foundation of the Easy Sleep technique. Therefore, adapting the technique to particular insomnia problems is quite simple. If you want to focus your practice on a specific sleeping goal, you just direct your imagination more specifically on that goal. As I now discuss adapting the technique to the four most common insomnia problems, you'll see what I mean. I'll also include some additional suggestions which may be of help to you along the way.

If Falling Asleep Is the Big Problem

Relax your muscles according to the basic unwinding instructions.

In Step Two (Directing), be sure your imaginary scene includes picturing yourself *falling asleep easily and effort-lessly*, as well as seeing yourself sleeping efficiently and awakening refreshed.

In Step Three (Drifting), add plenty of sensory detail, such as sounds, fragrances, feelings, colors, and movement. Imagine feeling more and more relaxed, more and more at peace with yourself and the world as you Drift through the scene. If, by chance, the imagined scene doesn't feel good enough, change it. For instance, suppose you're in the middle of an imaginary beach scene, and you find you just aren't in the beach mood. Try a different kind of scene, such as an indoor scene, a winter scene, a spring evening scene. Don't try hard to get exactly the right scene—just Drift into different ones until you find the scene of least resistance—then go with it.

Be sure you make use of the eye-roll procedure whenever you find your concentration wandering off your practice and onto those excitatory thoughts that keep you up.

If Awakening during the Night Is the Big Problem

Practice Steps One and Three according to the basic instructions.

When you get to Step Two (Directing), emphasize picturing yourself sleeping efficiently *through* the night. Although you will also imagine yourself awakening, feeling refreshed in the morning, your primary focus should be on imagining yourself sleeping throughout the night with all your energy systems maintaining their necessary balances.

With practice, you will be able to break this disturbing awakening pattern. However, in the meantime, if you should awaken in the "middle of the night," repeat the three steps of the technique to get back to sleep.

If Getting Up Too Early Is the Big Problem

Practice Steps One and Three according to the basic instructions.

During Step Two (Directing), your imaginary scene should emphasize awakening at the specific time you would like to wake up. If right now you are awakening two or more hours earlier than you desire, you might find it easier to start by imagining yourself getting up an hour later than usual. Once you have succeeded in extending your sleep by an hour, practice extending it another hour, and so on—until you are getting up at the time you'd like to.

If you should awaken in the morning before your desired time, repeat the three steps of the technique to go back to sleep.

If Unsound Sleep Is the Big Problem

Light or fitful sleep can also be specifically attacked during Step Two. Once you have relaxed your muscles (Step One), build your Directing scene around sleeping soundly and awakening feeling refreshed and rejuvenated. You might wish to imagine your self-awareness energy circuits turning down to a "low volume" for the night, turning back up as morning approaches, and arriving at their alert "ON" position when it's wake-up time.

After completing Step Two, go on to Step Three according to the general instructions.

If You Have More than One of the Big Four

First of all, you are not unique. Many who complain of light sleep also complain of getting up too early; many who have difficulty falling asleep also experience interrupted sleep; many who complain of having any one of the common insomnia problems also complain of having other ones occasionally.

If you do have more than one of the problems, develop your Step Two (Directing) scene accordingly. In other words, instead of building your scene around one major sleeping goal, build it around two or more goals. There are no limits. You can imagine yourself falling asleep easily AND sleeping through the night AND sleeping soundly AND awakening when you want to. Whatever sleeping problems you have, imagine yourself sleeping as if you didn't have them. Your brain will get the message.

What If . . .

By now, you should have a pretty good "book sense" of why and how the Easy Sleep concentration technique works. When you actually lie down to practice it, however, you will inevitably encounter some of those "what if" questions. There is a strong association link between facing something new and encountering "what if's." And it's certainly not a bad link to have in certain situations. It can protect you from investing in orange groves in Alaska or opening your front door before finding out who's on the other side of it. I will now answer some of the common "what if" questions related to the Easy Sleep technique.

1. *"What if my muscles always feel tight and I can't relax?"*
You *can* relax your muscles. To prove this to yourself, clench your fist tightly, then release the tension in your hand.

This little demonstration should convince you that you

have some degree of control over muscular tension. Through your practice of the Easy Sleep technique, that degree of control will increase and your ability to relax will improve.

2. *"What if I fall asleep before I get to Step Two or Step Three of the technique?"*

If falling asleep has been your major sleep problem, don't feel you have to force yourself to stay awake in order to "finish" your practice. The experience of falling asleep easily will strengthen your new expectation that you *can* fall asleep. Your *can sleep imprint* will thus be reinforced by the experience.

If your problem is awakening during the night, awakening too early, or unsound sleep, then begin your practice a few minutes earlier than your usual bedtime so you can complete Steps One and Two of the technique. If you still find yourself falling asleep the minute your head hits the pillow, practice Steps One and Two in a chair and get into bed for Step Three. If you happen to awaken at an undesirable hour, repeat the practice steps to return to sleep.

3. *"What if I can't roll my eyes up?"*

To demonstrate to yourself that you *can* roll your eyes upward, sit in a chair and look straight ahead; without moving your head up, roll your eyes toward the ceiling; then keeping your eyes in that position, close your lids.

During your practice at night, you may at first feel a little strain when you roll your eyes up, but that's because you are thinking so intensely, so much of the time. Eyes are in the "straight ahead" position during intense thinking activities. Until you are accustomed to the new eye position, just roll your eyes up momentarily at the beginning of your practice. If your thoughts become distracted during your practice, repeat the eye roll.

4. "What if my practice is interrupted for some reason?"

If your practice is interrupted by the ringing of a telephone or by some other disruption, handle the interruption calmly. When you return to your bed, you have the option of starting the technique over again or continuing on from where you were.

5. "What if I find it difficult to imagine myself sleeping efficiently during the Directing phase (Step Two) of the technique?"

Refer to the answers you gave to Question 19 in the sleep questionnaire (see Chapter 5). Then try constructing your imaginary Directing scene around one of those past experiences. Each time you practice the technique, you will become more proficient at using your imagination. However, if *picturing* a scene continues to be difficult for a while, then *say* the scene to yourself. For example, if you can't see yourself sleeping comfortably, then say to yourself, "I am sleeping comfortably. . . ." Both verbal suggestions and visual images leave imprints on your brain.

6. "What if I can't think of a Drifting scene for Step Three?"

Refer to the answers you gave to Question 20 in the sleep questionnaire (see Chapter 5). Your responses to that question should give you some good ideas. Again, with a little practice, those Drifting scenes will come easily.

7. *"What if I just can't concentrate during my practice?"*
Loosen your tongue! Roll your eyes! Take a few deep breaths to help you get relaxed, and don't try too hard to concentrate! The harder you try and the more determined you get, the more you will be "splitting" your energy. So take it easy. Since you are capable of reading, writing, speaking, and thinking, you can be sure you possess the ability to concentrate. You just need a little practice using your concentration abilities in this new, relaxed way.

8. *"What if I only have insomnia in certain situations? Should I still practice the technique every night?"*
Yes. Simply Direct your imagination to sleeping better in any and all situations. The more you practice the technique, the easier it will become for you to sleep in those "certain situations." Furthermore, the anxiety associated with those situations will decrease with practice.

9. *"What if the reason I awaken so early is that I really only require a small amount of sleep?"*
If you are satisfied with the sleep you're now getting and if you feel refreshed during the day, it's doubtful that you would want to bother changing your sleeping pattern. I assume that you are reading this book because you are dissatisfied with your sleeping pattern. If you are now awakening at 4 or 5 A.M. and would prefer to awaken at 6 or 7 A.M., there is no reason why you shouldn't be able to

extend your sleep by a few hours. If you follow the suggestions and instructions in this book, and if you begin to expect that you can sleep later, you'll find it relatively easy to adjust your sleep pattern.

10. "What if I want to stay up later at night and awaken later in the morning? I always fall asleep at about 10 P.M. and get up at about 4 A.M."

You can, of course, go to sleep at your present bedtime and awaken a few hours later by practicing the technique as described in this chapter. But, let's say you'd prefer to go to sleep at midnight and awaken at 8 A.M. First of all, you should be sure to include your new bedtime goal in your Directing scene. Imagine yourself going to bed later as well as getting up later. Secondly, you must begin to expect that you can stay up later, and it might be easiest if you started with a bedtime goal of 10:30 P.M. and gradually worked your way up to midnight. It's easier to expect that you can stay up a half-hour longer than two hours longer, and by succeeding a half-hour at a time, your expectation of success will grow stronger. Finally, you should be sure to follow the suggestions in Chapter 8, regarding daytime energy conservation.

11. "What if I find it necessary to take a sleeping medication occasionally?"

There is nothing wrong with taking an occasional sleeping pill or tranquilizer under your doctor's direction if the need should arise. In conjunction with the medication, however, be sure to practice the Easy Sleep technique. Through continued practice of the technique, your need for taking such medications in the future will diminish.

12. *"What if I am 'hooked' on sleeping pills?"*

As I stated earlier in this book, gradual withdrawal from the medication under your doctor's supervision is recommended. Practice the Easy Sleep technique in conjunction with your withdrawal program, or even before you start withdrawal from the medication. During Step Two (Directing), imagine yourself sleeping satisfactorily without the pills and feeling very good in the morning. Your practice will help to minimize or eliminate the undesirable effects sometimes associated with withdrawal from drugs. Once you are off the pills, continue practicing the technique.

13. *"What if I practice the Easy Sleep technique and it doesn't work?"*

It works. Reread or review the first six chapters of this book. The first time you read the material, you may have been preoccupied wondering what all that information had to do with *solving* your problem. Now that you know what the technique is, you can reread the material with a clearer perspective as to how it all contributes to the solution you're looking for. This second reading will enhance your expectations and your results considerably. So, look it over with a fresh perspective and keep practicing! Your sleep will improve!!!

* * *

The Easy Sleep concentration technique is your practical "how-to" for sleeping *when, where, how,* and *how much* you choose. It's your primary tool for instituting desirable changes in your present sleeping habits. But remember: The only way the technique works is by using it regularly. However, I'm sure you'll find that practicing the three steps will be a pleasant as well as effective way to use your energy.

As you begin practicing the Easy Sleep technique, you can make it ever easier on yourself if you also do a little complementary daytime planning. The next chapter will show you how to plan for better brain efficiency during the day, and consequently, better sleep at night.

8.

THE EASY SLEEP COMPANION: DAYTIME ENERGY CONSERVATION

New insomnia patients who come to see me seldom have difficulty describing their problem, its duration, its characteristics. Nor do they find it difficult to tell me how their sleeping problem makes them feel: "tired," "nervous," "unenthusiastic," "unmotivated," "rotten," "like a dish rag."

The difficulty arises when they are faced with this question during our initial interview: "If your sleeping problem were solved, what would you be able to do that you can't do now?" Their answer is inevitably something like this: "I'd feel better—I'd be more energetic."

That kind of response, however, does not answer the

question. The question is, "What would you *do?*" . . . NOT, "How would you *feel?*" While I don't mean to underestimate the value of feeling better—that's actually what you and everyone else wants most of all—I am trying to go just one step further. If you did feel better, the underlying implication is that you would *also* be able to *do better, do more, do something different* from what you are now doing.

Understandably, it's tough to answer the question, "What would you do if your sleeping problem were solved?" It's like answering the question: "If you had time on your hands to do anything you wanted to do, what would you do?" It's hard to come up with a response because you're so used to *not* being able to do anything you want to do, you seldom realistically consider an alternative. When you have a sleeping problem, you are caught in a similar bind. You are so used to *not* having enough energy that you hardly bother to think about what you would do if you did have enough energy.

But if you're going to solve your sleeping problem effectively and expediently, you *must* start thinking about what you'll do with the extra energy you'll gain as a result of your accomplishment. Even if you're just starting to use the Easy Sleep concentration technique—even though your sleeping problem is not yet solved—you must start making some plans for using that energy your insomnia has been depriving you of for so long. And, once you've made the plans, you must start instituting them. It's absolutely essential that you start this planning now, and that you institute the plans as soon as they're made.

The Necessity for Planning

At the present time, insomnia is depleting you of a certain amount of energy you undoubtedly could use during your daily life. Inadvertently, your daily energy supply is drained even further as you focus your awareness and concern on your sleeping problem. Naturally, you don't choose to use your energy in this self-defeating manner. It's an automatic human response. That is, when something troubles you, you tend to think about it. And thinking about a problem consumes energy.

What sort of energy-draining thoughts might you be engaging in during your waking life? There are three possibilities:

1) Thinking about the problem or change that interfered with your sleep in the first place. This category would include these kinds of thoughts:
- "Will I make a good impression at the board meeting? I've got to be sure I say the right thing."
- "Will my back ever stop bothering me?"
- "Without my husband (wife, mother, father, lover, children), life is empty."
- "Why did I volunteer for this job in the first place? I never learn my lesson."
- "The thought of moving again is making me sick."
- "I don't know what I'll do if I don't get accepted in graduate school."

2) Thinking about your sleep problem itself. For example:
- "I never get enough sleep."

- "No one in my family could possibly understand what I go through every night."
- "I haven't slept well in weeks. I hope tonight will be different ... but I know it really won't be."
- "I can't sleep."
- "Why can't I sleep?"
- "I'll never be able to sleep."

3) Thinking about the ramifications of your lack of sleep. For instance:
- "By five o'clock this afternoon, I'll be so drowsy, I won't be able to drive home."
- "By Friday, I won't be able to move a muscle."
- "I'll probably collapse in the middle of my final exams."
- "How in the world am I ever going to play in that golf tournament Sunday? I don't feel like I have enough energy to do anything."

Every bit of daily energy you use thinking about problems related to your sleep robs you of some of the energy you'd like to have for other purposes. In addition, because such thinking during the day is linked by association to your sleep problem, it serves to constantly fortify your *can't sleep imprint*. Thus, day and night you unwittingly reinforce your expectation that you won't be able to sleep well, that your performance will suffer, that you'll go through life feeling tired and groggy.

It would be meaningless to tell you to stop using your daily energy in this inefficient, self-defeating manner. It would be as meaningless as telling you to stop worrying or stop being tense or stop being negative. If I'm going to advise you to stop thinking about your sleep problem during the day, I must also tell you how to stop. I must offer you a pleasant and practical substitution. And that's where the planning and the new activity come into the picture.

The mere process of planning a new activity distracts some of that self-awareness energy off of your *can't sleep imprint*. And as you become involved in the activity, you significantly strengthen your new expectations regarding your ability to direct desirable changes. By planning something new and doing something new, you shift energy off of the areas that reinforce and retrigger your sleep problem.

What if you were to practice the Easy Sleep technique without making any complementary change in your daily energy use? You might end up with a stalemate situation in which you would undo during the day what you had done during the night. In other words, through your nightly practice, you would successfully weaken your *can't sleep imprint*. But through your daily, self-defeating thinking, you would restimulate your *can't sleep imprint*. It's possible that through use of the Easy Sleep technique alone you could solve your insomnia problem. But it would take longer, and there's really no sense in trying your patience at this point. This book is aimed at offering you the fastest, easiest, and most practical solution to your insomnia problem. Planning and instituting a new activity facilitates that goal.

It facilitates an additional goal as well—maintaining your new habit of satisfying sleep once you've got it. Through regular practice of the Easy Sleep mini-technique (Chapter 9), you'll be able to keep your self-directed sleeping skills sharp. But, as an added benefit of becoming an Easy Sleeper, you'll have a lot of extra energy on your hands—energy you haven't had for a while. Since you'll already have planned and started a new activity, you'll know just how to use some of that extra energy.

It's common knowledge that people frequently fall back into old habits after they've managed to "kick" them. One reason why this so often happens is because once the habit is gone, people find themselves with a lot of new-found energy, and they don't know where to channel it; they're not prepared.

Take a smoker, for example: He finally quits the habit and suddenly he finds that he doesn't know what to do with his hands; he doesn't know what to do while he's drinking his coffee; he doesn't know what to do with all that energy he'd been using to buy cigarettes, light them, flick the ashes, inhale, exhale, and worry about his smoking. He's left with what could only be described as a lot of nervous energy. Hence, more often than not, he'll start smoking again, or he'll perhaps take up overeating as a substitute.

After you've solved your sleeping problem, you'll feel more energetic than you've felt in the past. But you won't be stuck in the position of having "nervous energy" on your hands. You'll have a desirable activity ready for channeling that extra energy.

Coming Up with a Plan

Your primary source for obtaining extra energy during the day, as well as good sleep at night, will be the Easy Sleep concentration technique. But even if you aren't yet a regular practitioner of the technique, you already have a little more energy at your disposal than you did before you opened this book. That energy has come from your new understanding. I'll explain:

First of all, by understanding how changes in your life have resulted in your sleep problem, you are no longer perplexed by all those "why, why, why" questions. Secondly, by understanding how your thoughts can occur involuntarily, you no longer blame yourself for your inability to control them at night. Thirdly, by understanding how your previous attempts to solve your sleep problem failed despite your determination, you no longer feel responsible for your "failures." And finally, by understanding how you can gain control in an area where you couldn't before, you are no longer working against your old expectations of failure. Your new understanding has freed some of the energy that was previously tangled up by confusion. Remember: everything takes up energy, and confusing thoughts take up more energy than reasonable thoughts.

So with this little bit of extra energy you now have, I want you to get a pencil and paper and answer the following questions.

1) If your present sleeping problem were solved, how would you feel during the day as a result? (e.g. happier, more confident, more alert, etc.)
2) Based on your answer to the previous question, if you now felt the way you just indicated, what changes *in your present routine* would result?
   a) I'd get my work done faster. I wouldn't waste so much time.

b) I wouldn't make so many careless mistakes.

c) I'd be more communicative, outgoing.

d) I'd be able to concentrate on what I'm doing.

e) I wouldn't take so many naps.

f) It wouldn't take me so long to get going.

g) Other.

3) If the changes you indicated in 1 and 2 were now actualities, what *new activity or interest* could you pursue that is *not now part of your regular routine?*

a) I'd learn how to play golf (tennis, bridge, chess, etc.).

b) I'd start looking for a new job.

c) I'd go back to school.

d) I'd take a "self-improvement" course.

e) I'd start reading all those books I've always wanted to read.

f) I'd get involved in community affairs.

g) I'd start entertaining people at my home.

h) I'd start painting (sculpting, writing, etc.).

i) I'd invent something.

j) I'd become a film buff.

k) I'd become a gourmet cook.

l) Other.

As you begin to solve your sleeping problem, you *will* start feeling the way you indicated in Question 1. By virture of feeling more energetic, you will also find yourself becoming more efficient at carrying out your present routine, as indicated in Question 2. Your answer to Question 3, however, must stand out as something *entirely different* from your responses to 1 and 2. It is not sufficient to answer

Question 3 like this: "I'd spend more time with my family," or "I'd be able to improve my golf game." Those are Question 2 answers. You must pick out a *new* activity—one that you are not presently engaged in!

When should you select a new activity? Now, if possible. If you have to think about it for a while, think about it. Write down the possibilities and mull them over. Eliminate the ones that don't appeal to you, and then grab one that does. Don't hem and haw for days about what you can or can't do or what you REALLY want to do. It's a waste of energy. Just write down your ideas and MAKE A DECISION.

Once you have made your decision, you should immediately begin planning the new activity. Since you are already developing a new, reasonable expectation that your sleeping problem will be solved, PLAN THE ACTIVITY AS IF YOUR PROBLEM WERE ALREADY SOLVED. Use your imagination and pretend a little if you have to. Pretend you are the kind of sleeper you're going to be, and make the plans.

What does this planning entail? It depends on the activity you have selected. But to give you an idea of what your planning might include, here are some possibilities:

1) Determining how much the activity will cost and adjusting your budget accordingly.
2) Determining what supplies you'll need and how they can be obtained.
3) Obtaining schedules, informational materials, enrollment applications.

4) Talking to other people who are involved in the activity.
5) Going to the library for information or books on the subject.
6) Organizing a time schedule for yourself.
7) If you are convalescent or otherwise unable to obtain your own books or supplies, contact a service organization or friend who will help you.

Starting In

As soon as you have completed your preparations, begin *doing* your new activity. The more you practice the Easy Sleep concentration technique, the easier it will be for you to carry out your new daily plans. But don't wait until your sleeping problem is solved to start your activity. START IN AS IF YOUR PROBLEM WERE ALREADY SOLVED. The new activity will distract some of that energy off your *can't sleep imprint,* and it will prevent you from reinforcing your sleep problem during your waking hours.

If you are faced with a time gap between preparing for your new activity and beginning it—for example, if you have enrolled in a course that won't begin for a few months —do some related research or reading to stimulate your interest in the subject. You could also visit museums, classes, or other places to give you some background experience relative to your new activity. The point is: DO SOMETHING AS SOON AS POSSIBLE, AND KEEP IT UP.

Once you begin planning and instituting your new activity, there is always the possibility that you may decide the activity is just not for you. If this should happen, don't resign yourself to doing nothing. Be flexible and pick another activity. There is absolutely nothing wrong with trying many new and different things. On the contrary, with your new positive perspective about your ability to change, you can derive just as much benefit from sampling a number of activities as you can from pursuing one interest alone. So if the activity you select needs a replacement, sit down with your pencil and paper and make a new list of possibilities. Then—just as you did the first time—MAKE A DECISION, MAKE THE PLANS . . . and START IN!!!!

By complementing your nightly practice of the Easy Sleep technique with your new daily activity, you will have a 24-hour program aimed at better brain energy efficiency. You'll get maximal results from Easy Sleep within a minimal amount of time.

9.

THE
MINI-TECHNIQUE
FOR MAINTENANCE

Through understanding, practice, and daytime planning, you will have acquired the skill of self-directed sleep. Like any skill you master, this one must be exercised regularly to be kept in tune.

So, *after you have obtained a month of insomnia-free nights*, using the basic Easy Sleep concentration technique (see Chapter 7), you'll be ready to move on to the mini-technique: a streamlined practice tool for keeping your sleeping skill in good condition.

The Easy Sleep mini-technique serves a two-fold purpose: 1) It enables you to maintain your habit of satisfying, efficient sleep once you've got it; 2) It enables you to adapt smoothly to potentially sleep-disruptive situations, such as time-zone changes, hospital stays, and job schedule shifts. (We'll talk more about these common "sleep spoilers" in the next chapter.)

Instructions for practicing the mini-technique follow:

Before You Begin

Pre-Sleep Expectations:

By the time you start using the mini-technique, you should be approaching bedtime with a strong expectation of sleeping easily and efficiently. This expectation is based on your practical understanding of the principles of self-directed sleep, as well as your positive experience in having accomplished your goals. Thus, getting a good night's sleep is both plausible *and predictable* for you. Your expectations are now working for you every night.

Preparations:

The mini-technique is practiced in bed *every* night. Before practice, adjust your surroundings by reducing exterior distractions, just as you did with the basic Easy Sleep technique. You needn't allow extra time or make special provisions so that you can "complete" the technique before falling asleep. Such provisions may have been necessary when you were using the basic technique to solve particular problems (see Chapter 7, "What If . . ." #2), but they are no longer necessary. Since you don't have your old problem any more, it's perfectly all right if you get to sleep before Steps Two or Three of the mini-technique.

Your practice position with the mini-technique is optional. You can either practice on your back with your head elevated, or you can practice the whole technique in your usual sleeping position. The main point is to get comfortable before closing your eyes.

The Steps

Step One: Instant Unwinding

Now that you are experienced at unwinding your muscles with ease and control, you can achieve the same relaxed state by giving yourself a one-word signal. When you're in your comfortable position with your eyes closed, roll your eyes up momentarily and say the word "UNWIND" to yourself.

As you say this word, you will feel that excess tension and tightness uncoiling from your muscles. A deep feeling of relaxation will then spread from head to toe.

The reason a one-word signal can now be substituted for the gradual Unwinding procedure is because of your brain's imprint association capacity. Through those 30-plus days of practice with the basic Easy Sleep concentration technique, you have developed a strong association link between the word "UNWIND" and the feeling of relaxation elicited by the *unwinding* process. Thus, by repetition of the experience, you now have the capacity to take a shortcut—a single word, rather than a whole process, can now signal the desired reaction.

There is nothing magical, by the way, about the word "UNWIND." You can use a word such as "RELAX," or any other word, as long as it gives you the result you're looking for. Whatever *works best* for you *is best* for you.

Step Two: Instant Directing

After you unwind, you are ready to Direct your concentrated energy on a sleeping goal instantly. What you will Direct it on is *the time you wish to awaken in the morning.* In essence, during Step Two, all you do is "set your built-in alarm clock."

For example, if you want to wake up at 7 A.M., either *picture* yourself awakening at that time, or *tell* yourself to awaken at that time, or *imagine* yourself setting your own built-in alarm clock.

The Instant Directing step can be thought of as a brain-energy approach to putting in your own wake-up call. What you're doing is pre-programming yourself for the time you wish to arise.

Remember to set your "alarm" later on weekends or days off. With a little practice, you'll become quite adept at controlling your built-in clock; your precision may even surprise you at first. But's it's really no trick: you are, after all, the one who's directing the events.

Step Three: Drifting

The Drifting phase is the only activity that is performed the same way in both the mini-technique and the basic Easy Sleep concentration technique. So, imagine yourself in the midst of a comfortable, soothing, pleasantly monotonous situation. Drift through your imaginary scene, and it will lead right into sleep.

*   *   *

The mini-technique is designed for the "graduate" Easy Sleeper. In terms of activity and time, it's the basic Easy

Sleep concentration technique in its most abridged form. The Unwinding phase is condensed to only one word. The Directing phase is reduced to only one brain-energy focal point—the time you wish to awaken.

And, although the Drifting activity remains the same, the time required for this phase becomes minimal. The reason the Drifting activity is unchanged is because the onset of sleep is always facilitated by imagining something pleasant, calming, or neutral. The alternative would be to imagine something unpleasant, uncalming, or excitatory— hardly conducive to sleep. However, it *will* take you less time to drift off to sleep, and the reason is: As a graduate Easy Sleeper, you will be experienced in using your imagination in a sleep-inducing manner. With that old *can't sleep* barrier removed, it's a foregone conclusion that drifting off to sleep will be quick and easy.

The first two steps of the mini-technique can thus be completed in a minute or two. The third step doesn't have an actual completion point. It just leads naturally into sleep by facilitating the inhibitory process. However, the fact that sleep occurs naturally during Step Three (Drifting) in no way diminishes the fact that you have self-directed it. *You* are the one who establishes that controlled environment in your imagination. *You* are the one who concentrates your brain energy and directs it toward that desired result.

Once again, here are the steps of the mini-technique:

1) Instant Unwinding: With your eyes closed, momentarily roll them up beneath your lids; then say the word "UNWIND" (or another word of your choosing).

2) Instant Directing: Set your built-in "alarm clock" for your desired wake-up time.

3) Drifting: Imagine yourself in a comfortable, sensually satisfying, pleasantly monotonous scene.

The mini-technique *is* as easy as 1 . . . 2 . . . 3. It's the quickest, simplest way of keeping your self-directed sleeping skills in top condition.

Tailoring Your Maintenance

What if you feel a little more tense than usual on some nights? What if you want to focus your concentrated energy on a goal other than awakening at a certain time? Can the mini-technique be altered or expanded? Of course it can.

Here are some possibilities for tailoring your nightly maintenance, if the need should arise:

Altering Step One

If a one-word signal such as "UNWIND" doesn't evoke the degree of relaxation you desire, don't be discouraged. No one goes to bed with exactly the same degree of muscular tension every night.

When you first make the shift from the basic concentration technique to the mini-technique, it *may* happen that one word isn't sufficient for you. You may just need a little more practice relaxing your muscles. You may just need to build up a stronger association link between your word-signal and your desired muscular response.

On the other hand, if you've been using the one-word

signal successfully but you then experience a night when your signal doesn't produce the desired result, you may just be a bit more tense than usual. In most instances, this tension is related to some stressful activity you have experienced during the day. You may need a little more time to Unwind.

So, if at any time the one-word signal doesn't produce the desired result, feel free to add more words such as "Unwind . . . Let go . . . Feel the tension uncoiling and fading away." Or, if you prefer, you can give yourself the one-word signal and then selectively Unwind a particularly tight group of muscles. You can also start your basic Unwinding exercise, relaxing your muscles group by group from the top of your head down to a point such as your shoulders; then, from your shoulders, you can use your imagination to "drive" that relaxation right down to your toes.

In summary, if one word doesn't do the Unwinding job sufficiently, take a little more time and embellish the step according to your own needs. You can't overdose on the Easy Sleep technique.

Altering Step Two

In the mini-technique, the only Step Two activity I have specified is "setting your built-in alarm clock," or "putting in your wake-up call." This brief Directing step serves to reinforce your control over awakening when you want to. It's the kind of control that comes in quite handy if you ever want to readjust your sleeping schedule. In addition, by Directing yourself to get up at a certain time, you are much more likely to awaken feeling refreshed and ready (as opposed to feeling like you've been impolitely jolted from deepest sleep).

However, if you want to give yourself a few more messages or expand upon your "wake-up" message, go right ahead. For example, if you want to awaken an hour or two earlier than your usual time (to catch a plane, etc.), you may wish to take a few extra minutes to Direct your imagination on awakening early *and* feeling refreshed and unhurried in the morning. Or, suppose you are one of those people who long ago acquired the skill of awakening any time you choose? If you happen to be among the population who never has to rely on clock radios or alarms, during your practice of the mini-technique you may prefer to take a minute or two to Direct your energy on feeling energetic and revitalized in the morning.

Since you are the "director," you can use Step Two to reinforce or to direct any sleeping/waking message you would like. With your old insomnia problem out of the way, you have a golden opportunity to branch into new areas of self-directed sleep and to make any improvements you desire.

Lifetime Tools

The basic Easy Sleep concentration technique is your main tool for solving your sleep problem. The mini-technique is your means for keeping your self-directed sleeping skills sharp and precise for the rest of your life.

You should not, however, forget about that new daytime activity you instituted in conjunction with your practice. Not only does the activity help you change your old sleep habits, but it also gives you an added sense of your own potentials and flexibility. So by all means keep up that spirit of exploration; continue to develop new interests and activities; continue to try new and different things which appeal to you.

Remember, better brain efficiency night and day can only make you feel better night and day. Through ongoing use of the Easy Sleep approach, an energy saving approach, you can continually add new dimensions to your life—AT YOUR OWN DIRECTION.

10.

FOILING THE SLEEP SPOILERS

One of the ongoing advantages of self-directed sleep is that you can apply your skills to any potentially disruptive sleeping situation you ever encounter. Even those good sleepers out there who have never considered themselves "real insomniacs" usually wind up helpless in certain "sleep spoiling" situations. But not so for you. As an experienced Easy Sleeper, you'll be well-prepared to deal with the realities of living in a world that is not always conducive to sleep.

In this chapter, I'll offer you some guidelines and tips for foiling the common "sleep spoilers."

Spoiler #1: The Time Lag

You take a 9 P.M. flight out of New York and arrive in Rome eight hours later. But somewhere between New York and Rome, you lose five hours. It's 10 A.M. in Rome when you land, and as much as you'd like to do as the Romans do, it's not easy when your body feels like 5 o'clock in the morning, Eastern Standard Time.

You're a nurse, and you've just been informed that you'll be required to work the night shift every fourth week. How can you make the transition from the day shift to the night shift and back again smoothly?

Whether you're crossing time zones in the air or changing time schedules on the ground, you're essentially confronting the same kind of situation—the "lag" situation. What the "lag" means is that your biological clock is out of phase with the clock on the wall. Although your body has the capacity to conform to a new schedule, it requires a certain period of adjustment to reset itself. Unfortunately, the clock on the wall waits for no one.

Why is this adjustment time necessary? Years of research by biologists and other scientists clearly show that all living creatures possess internal biological rhythms. In humans as well as in other mammals, this so-called "biological clock" revolves around periods of approximately 24 hours. Or, to state it another way, our many internal functionings follow a "circadian rhythm" ("circa" meaning "around," "dies" meaning "day").

"In man," explains Dr. William C. Dement of Stanford University, "more than one hundred functions and structural elements can be named which oscillate between maximal and minimal values once a day. They range from the well-known rhythm in deep body temperature to rhythms in mood and mental performance."[1]

Thus, within a basic 24-hour period, every biochemical and physiologic function in your body maintains a regular rhythm of rest and activity ... of "highs" and "lows." All of these internal functions are paced in relationship to each other, and all are timed to synchronize with a 24-hour time cycle.

Your biological clock does not necessarily have to be set in the traditional breakfast-in-the-morning, lunch-at-noon, dinner-in-the-evening pattern. Nor does it have to be set in accordance with the light of day and the dark of night. The pattern of man's sleep, University of Florida psychologist Wilse B. Webb concludes, "appears dominantly to be a sleep of choice within reasonable limits and is more clock-bound than light bound in terms of cues."[2] Hence, biologically-speaking it's not particularly significant whether you sleep by night and work by day or vice versa. What does matter is that your living pattern adheres to a fairly regular 24-hour cycle of rest and activity.

In light of that information, let's now look at a typical jet lag situation. If your body's 24-hour cycle is synchronized with Eastern Standard Time, what happens when you fly to Rome and jump ahead five hours?

The usual result is that all of those internal, oscillating activities are still at the 5 A.M. (E.S.T.) point in their 24-hour biological cycle, although the clock in Rome is at the

10 A.M. point in its cycle. As a consequence, all sorts of little biological readjustments must take place to get your internal rhythms in gear with the new clock-time.

Changing work shifts can pose the same kind of challenge. If you've been working the 7 A.M. to 3 P.M. shift and suddenly you're required to work the 11 P.M. to 7 A.M shift, you may get stuck with a time-lag situation. At 4 A.M., you can be faced with a task you're accustomed to performing at noon. At 2 P.M. you can be faced with the prospect of going to sleep, an activity you're used to indulging in at 10 P.M.

Most people do manage to adapt to new time schedules eventually. However, for the person who doesn't know the principles and tools of self-directed sleep, this adaptation time can vary anywhere from one day to a few weeks, or more—such a person has no real control over how quickly and smoothly the adjustment is made. To add to his predicament, he may even *expect* to have problems adjusting. From his point of view, the so-called "jet-lag syndrome" might seem to be "inevitable." A person might also view his sleeping pattern as a non-changeable part of his "personality" (such as being a "born night owl" or an "inveterate lark").

As an experienced Easy Sleeper, you *do* have control over how quickly and smoothly you adjust to those "lag" situations. You can also expect to adapt easily to such circumstances. You have already successfully self-directed a change in your sleeping pattern, so you know you can do it again. You do not view your sleeping style as a fixed aspect of your personality.

Therefore, you can easily reset your biological clock to conform to a time change *within a day*. The *time* you usually go to sleep is, after all, an imprint. This imprint is linked by association to numerous other imprints—"feeling" imprints, "organic activity" imprints, "visual" imprints, and more. By using the Easy Sleep technique, you can readily direct your brain energy to form a new association link between the clock time and your bedtime. As a consequence, your numerous biological activities will get into phase by association.

I'll now offer you some suggestions for applying your self-directed sleeping skills to "lag" situations.

When your day is shortened by jet travel, as would happen if you flew from Los Angeles to Boston, or from New York to Rome, these tips are advised:

1) If you arrive early in the morning, but your body "says" it's even earlier, use your Easy Sleep technique to *take a nap*. Unwind your muscles as usual to get yourself relaxed (Step One); then Direct your imagination on awakening at a desired hour *in your new time zone* (Step Two); finally, Drift off to sleep (Step Three). The length of nap you choose will depend upon how early in the morning you arrived, how much sleep you obtained on the airplane, and how tired you feel. Whether you sleep for two hours or six hours, you should view this sleep as *a nap*, not as a "night's sleep."

2) If you arrive in the evening, but your body says it's still early, engage in some activity for a while. Have a late dinner; then use your Easy Sleep technique to go to sleep at the desired time *in the new time zone*. During the directing phase of your

practice (Step Two), imagine yourself awakening at the time you desire with all your body's internal activities synchronized to the appropriate clock-time.

When your day is lengthened by jet travel, as would happen if you flew from Boston to Los Angeles, or from Rome to New York, here are some pointers:

1) If you arrive early in the morning, but your body says it's later, use your technique to *take a nap* during the day. During Step Two of your practice, Direct your imagination to *awakening before the dinner hour in your new time zone*. After dinner, engage in some activity for a while; go to sleep that night at the appropriate hour, based on the new time. Always use the Easy Sleep technique to Direct yourself to sleep, of course.

2) If you arrive in the evening, but your body says it's later, have a snack if you're hungry. Then use your technique to Direct yourself to sleep efficiently and to awaken at the desired hour in the new time zone.

By the way, since you are skilled at self-directed sleep, you *can* use the Easy Sleep technique during your flight. Therefore, if you desire, you can start synchronizing your biological clock while in the air.

When you are faced with changing work shifts the suggestions for smooth adaptation are similar:

1) Take a nap prior to beginning your new work schedule. After you unwind (Step One), Direct your imagination to resetting your biological clock to conform to your new schedule.

2) Once you start on the new shift, use your technique before sleep to reinforce your synchronization.

The extent and character of "lag" posed by jet travel and schedule shifts cover a broad spectrum. Thus, the manner in which you use the Easy Sleep technique to adjust to the time changes—whether you use the technique to take a "synchronization nap" or to sleep for the night—will depend upon the circumstances. You always have the option to employ the basic Easy Sleep concentration technique or the mini-technique, expanding or tailoring the three steps to suit your own needs.

With your positive expectations of adjusting smoothly, and with your tools for making the adjustment you can easily synchronize your body-time with the clock-time in *a day. One day for synchronization* is well within *your capacity.*

Spoiler #2: Noises

The neighbor's kids are having a party, and if you didn't know better, you'd swear they had planted a guitar amplifier under your bed. "Boom, Boom, Bop, Bop . . ." the music goes on . . . and on . . . and ON. How can you possibly get to sleep? You feel like you're in the middle of a thunder storm.

You're just drifting off to sleep when your mate's snoring picks up volume and invades your reverie. You deliberately clear your throat—loudly. When that doesn't work, you give him (her) a little kick. You finally decide to take the big step and awaken him (her). The decision pays off—for a few minutes. The snoring starts up again, and this time you kick a little harder. You'd like to get some sleep, too! But, how?

Snoring partners and "inconsiderate" neighbors are but two of the many sounds that invade bedrooms. Living in a noise-infested world, we are surrounded by a barrage of horn-honking cars; revving motorcycles; television sets; air traffic, and occasional stereophonic, quadrophonic, electrophonic auditory insults.

As an Easy Sleeper, however, you have all the necessary equipment for filtering out most noise invaders.

As you know, excitatory thinking—that inability to shift one's awareness off of some past event, anticipated event, or incoming signal—is what keeps people awake. Once you have mastered the skills of self-directed sleep, you *have* the *ability* to shift your awareness off of whatever it is that's intruding upon your peaceful environment.

Whether it's a noisy party or a snoring partner that has caught your awareness when you want to go to sleep, there are some particularly relevant points you've learned from experience:

—The more energy you focus on the noise, the more disturbing the noise will become, and the more difficult it will be to fall asleep;

—Even without the tools of Easy Sleep, you'd *eventually* fall asleep from sheer exhaustion, noise or no noise;

—*With* the Easy Sleep technique, you know how to shift your thoughts off of wakeful signals; based on experience, you have an expectation that you *can* control the focus of your awareness.

When faced with a particularly noisy situation, you don't have to wait until you fall asleep from sheer exhaustion. Instead, use your practice technique to distract your awareness off of the noise. Here are some guidelines:

1) Take your time Unwinding (Step One). The more relaxed you are, the easier it will be to direct yourself to sleep.

2) Direct your imagination to sleeping efficiently throughout the night and awakening refreshed (Step Two). Use this step to build up your confidence a bit.

3) Incorporate the noise into your Drifting scene (Step Three). Through your imagination, make the noise a part of the background sound in your scenery. As you imagine the pleasing sensations of the scene, the background sound will fade further and further away.

4) If a noise should awaken you after you've fallen asleep, use your mini-technique to drift easily back to sleep.

Spoiler #3: Discomfort

The flu, a sunburn, a sprained ankle, heartburn, indigestion, a stuffy nose: these transient sources of discomfort can sometimes cause difficulty for the would-be sleeper. And, as everyone knows, pain and discomfort tend to feel worse at night.

Why this heightened discomfort at night? The situation is at least partially due to the increased amount of awareness we focus on the problem when we're in bed. Without the day's activities to distract us off our discomfort, we almost invariably find ourselves thinking more about our aches and pain.

In these situations, the Easy Sleep technique can be particularly valuable, not only as a means for obtaining a good night's sleep, but also as a mechanism for distracting our awareness off our discomfort. Here are some tips when discomfort threatens to spoil your sleep:

1) Take your time Unwinding, particularly if certain muscles feel tighter than usual.

2) As you Direct your energy to obtaining a good night's sleep, also imagine yourself awakening in the morning feeling much better.

3) Add plenty of sensory detail to your Drifting scene so it will provide you with maximum distraction. Also, choose your scene to fit your specific needs. For example, if you're chilled, you might imagine yourself in a warm summer scene. If you're uncomfortably warm, you might want to drift through a cool, refreshing winter scene.

Spoiler #4: The Big Day Is Tomorrow

The night before your big golf tournament; the night before an important exam; the night before you make your presentation to the board of directors: Anticipating a big event is a common "sleep spoiler." Often, the "spoiler" is made even worse by thoughts such as, "I've got to get a good night's sleep in order to do my best tomorrow."

First of all, you must understand that no amount of in-bed thinking is going to alter the next day's outcome. Second of all, you can rest assured that you have a certain reserve of energy that can help you "rise to that big occasion," even if you haven't had the "best" night's sleep in the world.

Thus, when the big day is tomorrow, you can still approach your sleep with a confident, casual attitude. Just keep these points in mind: 1) In-bed speculating will not change tomorrow's outcome; 2) Extra special sleep that night is not going to make you or break you.

With your casual attitude, you can then effectively employ your Easy Sleep technique to shift your awareness off the anticipated event and onto the steps leading to a good night's sleep.

In essence, when the big day is tomorrow, practice your Easy Sleep technique not with fervor, but with pleasure. If you assume a "so-what" attitude about your sleep, you'll make it even easier on yourself.

Spoiler #5: A Stay in the Hospital

Sleeping pills are almost routinely ordered for the majority of hospitalized patients.

The reasons for such standing orders are understandable. The hospital routine, first of all, tends to force a patient into a sleeping schedule which he isn't accustomed to. Second, the hospitalized patient often naps during the day, sometimes making it more difficult for him to fall asleep at bedtime. Third, the patient's worries and anxieties about his health can make it difficult for him to "let go" and sleep. From a medical point of view, adequate rest is always advisable for a patient. Thus, the well-intentioned sleeping pill is offered to aid the hospitalized individual.

Although hospitalization can disturb sleep in a variety of ways, you're at a definite advantage if you know the tools of self-directed sleep.

One advantage is that you can easily filter out external disruptions such as light and noise. Another advantage is that you have an insomnia-prevention tool, once you are released from the hospital. A further advantage is that you can adjust to a new time-schedule of sleeping and awakening.

For you, the only potential sleep "spoiler" posed by the hospital situation is the increased awareness energy you use in focusing your attention on your health problem. Excitatory thinking, agitated depression, and anxiety aren't always that easy to avoid when the bulk of your concern is occupied by your health.

However, if a stay in the hospital should become necessary, your positive, reasonable expectations will be working to enhance your results. What kind of positive expectations should you have? Here are some:

1) You should have an expectation of confidence regarding your doctor's knowledge and ability to help restore your health.

2) You should have an expectation that you can assist your doctor by obtaining a good night's rest.

3) You should have an expectation that your practice of the Easy Sleep technique is helping to establish and maintain a good energy balance, biochemically as well as emotionally.

During a hospital stay, these recommendations are also advised:

1) Use your Easy Sleep technique every night.

2) If you have any questions or problems, talk them over with your physician during the day. This will alleviate your tendency to excessively worry and wonder at night.

3) If you feel the need for the additional aid offered by a sleeping medication, then take the pill *in conjunction with your practice of the Easy Sleep technique.*

❋   ❋   ❋

Being human, you are not a perfectly consistent creature. You're not always content or always calm or always in control of your every thought and feeling. Problems, losses, worries, upheavals, and other significant changes, whether "good" or "bad," all affect you to some degree. It would, therefore, be ridiculous to assume that no matter what happens in your life, you'll drift pleasantly off to sleep every night.

This book is based on reasonable, realistic expectations. In the midst of some crisis in your life, it would be unreasonable to expect you to sleep with utmost efficiency every night and to awaken feeling invigorated every morning.

So, even after you have long since solved your insomnia problem and have graduated to the streamlined mini-technique, there may be occasional instances when sleeping is more difficult than usual. In such instances, you always have the option of using the full Easy Sleep concentration technique or expanding the mini-technique as you see fit. Through the creative use of your imagination, you have a lifetime tool that's adaptable to any sleeping situation. Once you discover the extent and versatility of your self-direction regarding sleep, the skill is yours forever.

11.

GOOD MORNING ...
EVERY MORNING

Although you have now completed this book, you are at a new beginning.

At one time, you may have thought your insomnia was a sign of some sort of psychological weakness.

At one time, you may have felt your sleeplessness wasn't a *real, physical* problem.

At one time, you may have thought your undesirable sleep patterns were beyond the realm of your own control.

Now, with your new understanding of what's going on "in your head," I hope you can view your sleep problem and all your problems as being real, physical recordings on your brain.

I hope you also understand that your sleeping difficulties were never your fault. Your inability to sleep was never a reflection of your lack of will power, your desire or your determination.

Insomnia develops when an individual has no practical tools for preventing it. And insomnia perpetuates itself when an individual has no tools for stopping it.

Now you have the tools. You not only can *solve* your present sleeping difficulties, but you can also *take charge* of your own sleeping/waking processes. You can change your sleep patterns or adjust them at any time in your life— *at your own direction.*

In addition, you can discover the advantages of having enough energy to approach each day with your eyes wide open. You can use your new-found energy to explore territory that had always seemed closed to you. You can try many new and different things. Getting through the day will no longer be the kind of struggle it once was. You will be among the energetic population.

To awaken each morning feeling alert, clear-headed, and refreshed is not an impossible dream. It's a benefit you're entitled to. It's also a benefit you can easily have, now that you know how to get it.

Good morning! Every morning!

NOTES AND REFERENCES

Chapter Notes

Chapter 1

1. Allan Rechtschaffen and Lawrence J. Monroe. "Laboratory Studies of Insomnia." *Sleep: Physiology and Pathology,* ed. A. Kales. Philadelphia: J. B. Lippincott Co., 1969.

Chapter 4

1. William C. Dement. *Some Must Watch While Some Must Sleep.* San Francisco: W. H. Freeman and Co., 1974.

2. Ivan P. Pavlov. "The Reflex of Purpose." *Lectures on Conditioned Reflexes.* New York: International Publishers Co., Inc., 1928.

3. Ibid.

Chapter 5

1. Ronald Kotulak, "Nice Guys Finish First in the Game of Longevity." *Chicago Tribune,* Oct. 10, 1976.

Chapter 10

1. William C. Dement. *Some Must Watch While Some Must Sleep.* San Francisco: W. H. Freeman and Co., 1974.

2. Wilse B. Webb. "Twenty-four-Hour Sleep Cycling." *Sleep: Physiology and Pathology,* ed. A. Kales. Philadelphia: J. B. Lippincott Co., 1969.

Other References

Feinberg, Irwin. "Effects of Age on Human Sleep Patterns." *Sleep: Physiology and Pathology,* ed. A. Kales. Philadelphia: J. B. Lippincott Co., 1969.

Foulkes, David. *The Psychology of Sleep.* New York: Charles Scribner's Sons, 1966.

Freemon, Frank R. *Sleep Research: A Critical Review.* Springfield: Charles C Thomas, 1972.

Hartmann, Ernest L., *The Functions of Sleep.* New Haven, London: Yale Univ. Press, 1973.

"In Pursuit of Sleep," *Town and Country Magazine,* March, 1977.

Kahn, Carol. "Do You Dream (Perchance) of Sleeping?". *Family Health,* Sept. 1977.

Kleitman, Nathaniel. *Sleep and Wakefulness.* University of Chicago Press, 1963.

Linde, Shirley Motter. *The Sleep Book.* New York: Harper & Row/Collins Associates Book, 1974.

Luce, Gay Gaer and Segal, Julius. *Sleep.* New York: Coward–McCann, Inc., 1966.

———. *Insomnia.* Garden City, N.Y.: 1969.

Magoun, Horace W. *The Waking Brain.* (2nd edition). Springfield: Charles C Thomas, 1963.

Ullrich, Polly. "Mister Sandman, Make Me A Dream." *Chicago Daily News,* Aug. 13–14, 1977.

U.S. Institute of Mental Health. *Current Research on Sleep and Dreams.*